J[illegible]n

CLEAN & LEAN DIET

THE INTERNATIONAL BESTSELLING BOOK ON ACHIEVING YOUR PERFECT BODY

James Duigan, world-renowned wellness guru and owner of Bodyism, London's premier health and wellness facility, is one of the world's top personal trainers. Bodyism's glittering client list includes Elle Macpherson, Rosie Huntington-Whiteley, David Gandy, Holly Valance, and Hugh Grant. He is also the author of the bestselling *Clean & Lean Flat Tummy Fast!*, *Clean & Lean Diet Cookbook*, and *Clean & Lean Warrior*.

with Maria Lally

KYLE BOOKS

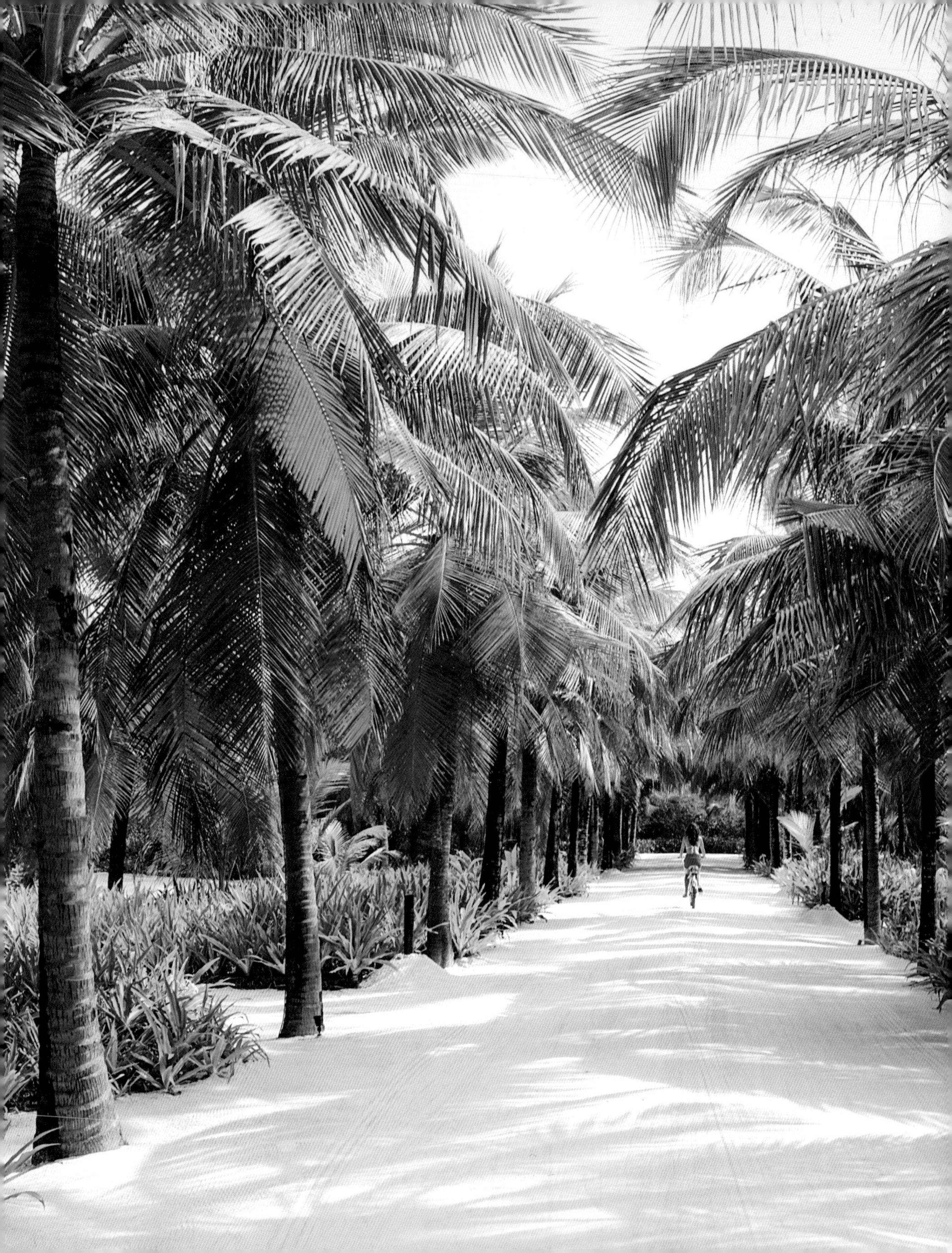

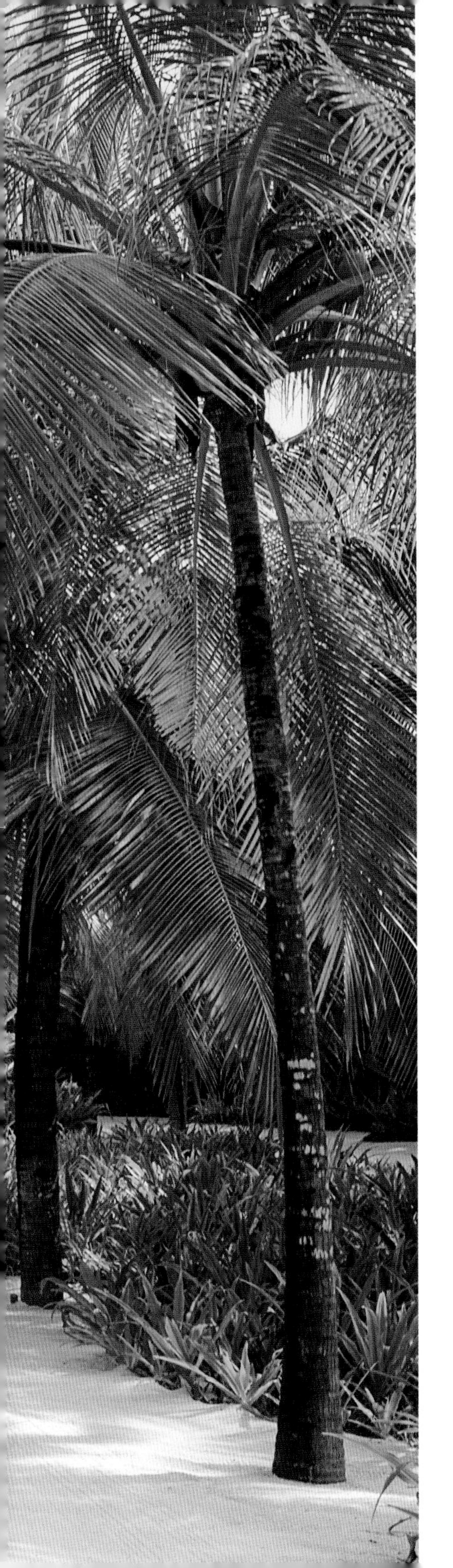

James Duigan

CLEAN & LEAN DIET

THE INTERNATIONAL BESTSELLING BOOK ON ACHIEVING YOUR PERFECT BODY

James Duigan

with Maria Lally

Photography by Sebastian Roos and Charlie Richards

Shot on location at the

One & Only Resorts, Mauritius and Maldives

KYLE BOOKS

Published in 2013 by Kyle Books
www.kylebooks.com

Distributed by National Book Network
4501 Forbes Blvd., Suite 200
Lanham, MD 20706
Phone: (800) 462-6420
Fax: (800) 338-4550
Customercare@nbnbooks.com

First published in Great Britain in 2010 by
Kyle Cathie Limited

ISBN 978-1-909487-02-4

Editor Judith Hannam
Assistant editor Vicki Murrell
Design Dale Walker
Models Christiane Duigan, Nathalie Shyllert
Location styling Emilie Lind
Recipe home economy and styling Mima Sinclair
Copy editor Anne Newman
Production Lisa Pinnell

Library of Congress Control Number: 2013935549

Printed in China

The information and advice contained in this book are intended as a general guide. Neither the author nor the publishers can be held responsible for claims arising from the inappropriate use of any remedy or exercise regime. Do not attempt self-diagnosis or self-treatment for serious or long-term conditions before consulting a medical professional or qualified practitioner. Do not begin any exercise program or undertake any self-treatment while taking other prescribed drugs or receiving therapy without first seeking professional guidance. Always seek medical advice if any symptoms persist.

CONTENTS

{Foreword}
by Elle Macpherson

I met James in the mid-90s before I became pregnant with my first son. As I watched him train at the gym, where I was on the running machine, I was fascinated by his elegance and by his effortless exercising. He was lean and strong but not pumped up—he was focused and self-aware. I immediately wanted to work with him, as he seemed to have something I hadn't seen in other trainers.

We started working together and he immediately understood that I wanted to maintain a long, lean, healthy body while retaining my femininity and curves.

He also knew we didn't have the luxury of time or the headspace to be obsessive at the gym.

We worked on my body, attitude, diet, balance, strength, and consistency.

James' approach is non-gimmicky and straightforward. He works from the inside out—clearing the body and the mind and doing varied exercises. Soon I became in the best shape ever—mentally and physically.

We've been through a lot together over the last twenty years or so, including my second pregnancy, numerous photo shoots, and red carpet appearances. We're both Australian and we love an outdoor lifestyle.

A true testament to his workouts is that, twenty years on, we still train together because he keeps it relevant and fun—it works! There is literally nobody better in the world than James for getting a woman's body into amazing shape.

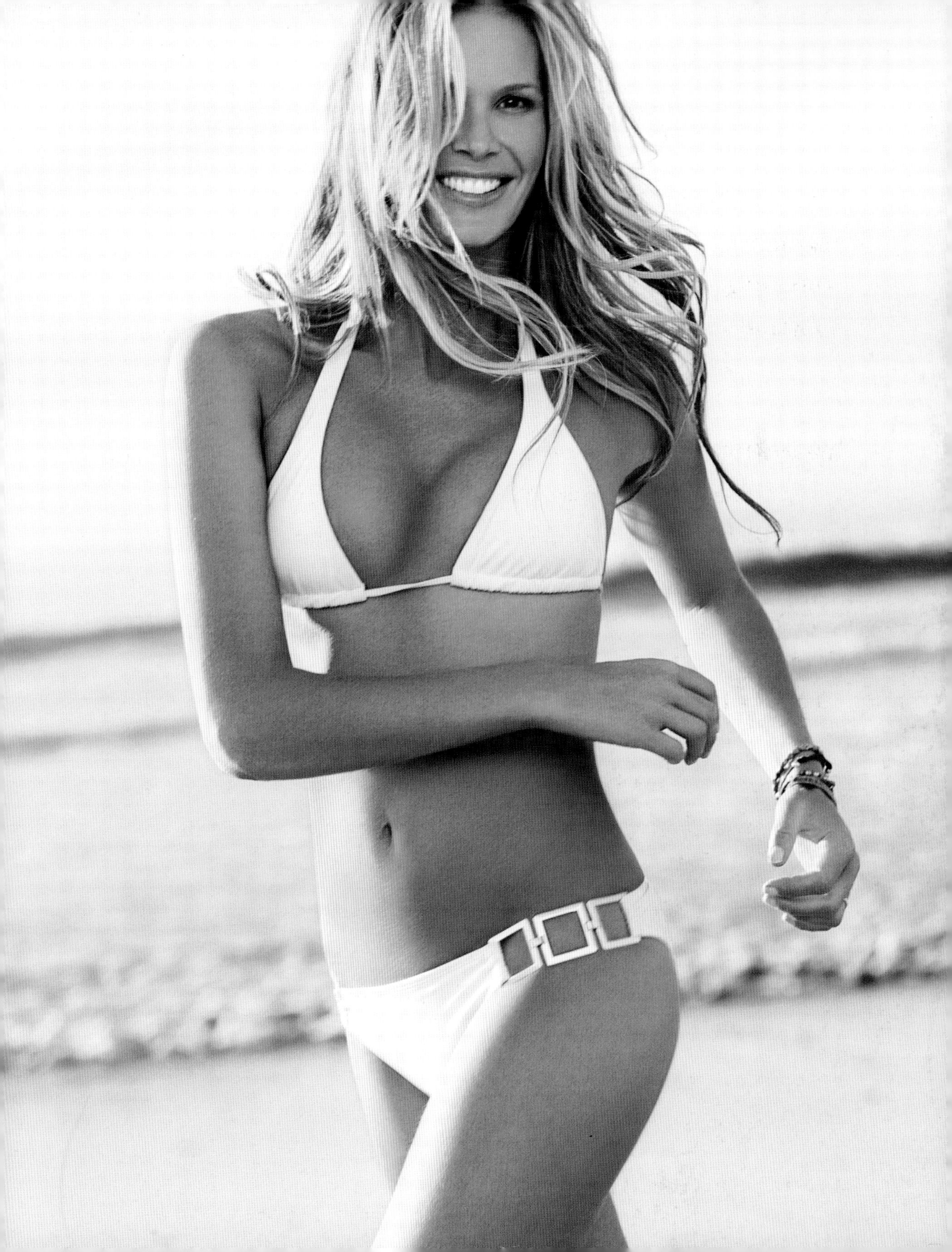

INTRODUCTION

I would like to start by saying thank you to everyone who has supported this book. It has been passed from sisters to daughters to husbands to brothers to friends and I am so grateful to all of you. Thank you for giving me the opportunity to change your life. When I wrote the first Clean & Lean book and it quickly became a bestseller worldwide, it was proof that my Clean & Lean philosophy can work for you. It has worked for hundreds of thousands of people all over the world from all walks of life—from workaholics to world travelers, to parents who have to hold down jobs while looking after children and running a home—and many have written to tell me how this book has changed their life. Clean & Lean can work for anyone. It's easy and achievable and I'm sure it will work for you.

First up, here's what you need to know: you deserve a happy, healthy, and fulfilled life. It may sound strange, and it breaks my heart, but many of us don't believe we deserve this. However, once you understand that you do, every choice you make to be healthy stops being a battle. Imagine that!

Any transformation that happens in your body, happens in your mind first. I want you to let go of shame and guilt and change the conversation you have with yourself. Be kind, be forgiving, and give yourself a powerful platform from which you can make these transformations. Remember, beautiful isn't how you look, it's how you feel. I think you're amazing for picking up this book, and it's about time you thought so too. Clean & Lean is based on self-acceptance and self-love. Once you have this, the rest is easy.

Now, here's the good news: your body really, really wants to be slim. It wants to be lean and light, strong and energized, simply because that's the way it's designed to be—lean and healthy is its natural state.

Don't believe the myth that the human body clings on to fat. It doesn't—because it knows that's not the way it functions best. However, when you eat or drink processed foods, alcohol, bad fats, and refined sugar your body becomes overloaded with toxins. It's these toxins, and not your body, that cling on to the fat.

But if your body looked the way it should—lean and light—you'd feel pretty amazing. People think it is normal to wake up feeling tired and grumpy, but it's not. It might be common, but it certainly isn't normal. Normal is waking up feeling clean and lean, rested, energized and ready to take on the day. When you get Clean & Lean you won't need sugar to help you function in the morning and you won't get that crashing tiredness in the afternoon that only more coffee or a chocolate cookie can (briefly) keep at bay.

Instead, you'll wake up after a good night's sleep, feeling refreshed. Your energy levels will be high, as will your concentration levels, sex drive, and mood. So your job now is to make the choice to take action and stick to it. And I'm going to show you how to do it: how to eat, how to exercise, and how to ensure that you stay motivated.

First off, it's important to understand that your weight and health are not separate issues. Being overweight is a symptom of being unhealthy. Focus on your health and the weight will drop off. You will also need to learn the difference between an excuse and a reason. Be brutally honest: if you really want something you'll find a way to get it.

Your health and happiness are important, so stand strong.

You must believe you can do this (you can, I know you can). It doesn't matter how often you have failed in the past—your past does not equal your future. What matters now is focusing on what you want, identifying what you need to get it, and taking consistent action. Your health and happiness are important, so stand strong. Create a support system for yourself. Ask your friends and family for help; if they choose not to encourage you, they may not be the best people to be around right now.

You don't have to follow every single rule religiously but stick wholeheartedly to those you can manage and you'll be blown away by the results. Enjoy your food, enjoy your life, tell someone that you love them, forgive yourself for everything, and get on with being an inspiration and the beautiful person that you are. Today. So now read on, follow each easy step and—like thousands before you—watch your body transform. I promise you, this works!

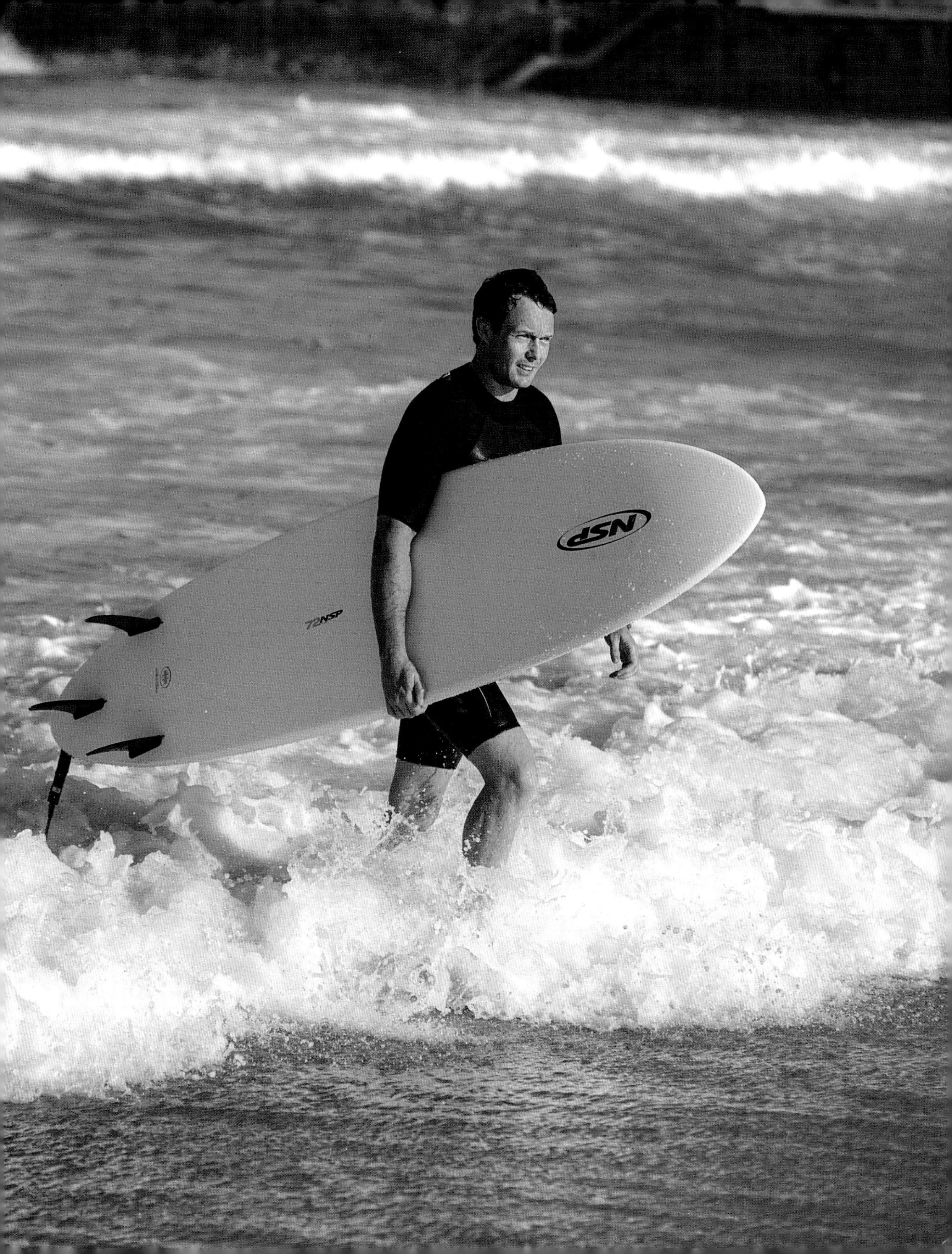
NSP
72NSP

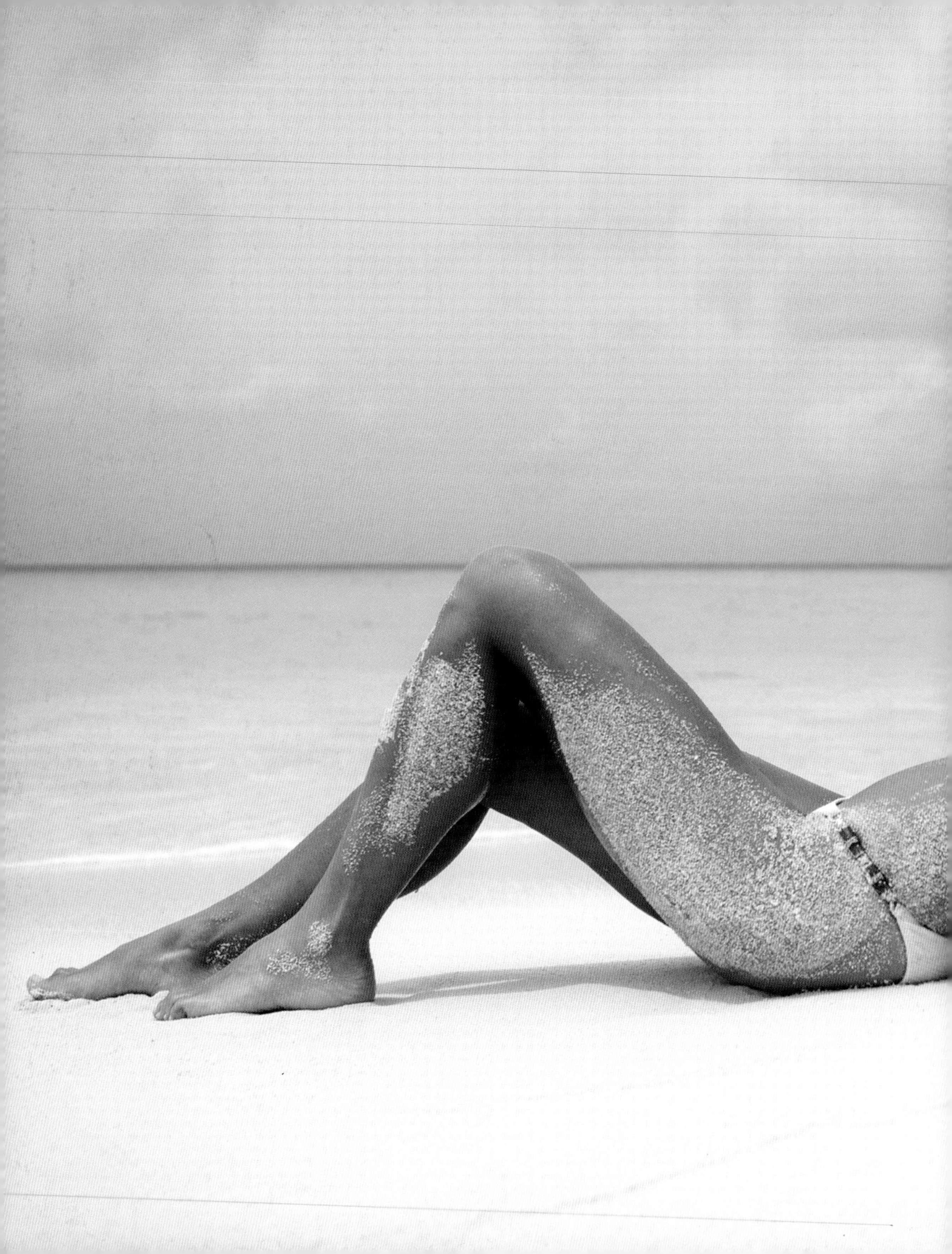

CHAPTER 1

WHY CLEAN EQUALS LEAN

THIS CHAPTER WILL REVEAL...

WHY DIETING IS A WASTE OF TIME

WHY TOXINS MAKE YOU FAT

HOW ORGANIC FOOD CAN HELP TO MAKE YOU SLIM

PART ONE

THE CLEAN SECTION

"Clean & Lean" is a term I came up with, which describes the ultimate approach to achieving the perfect body. The word "clean" here means a body that can deal effectively with toxins—one that can deal with the few that sneak in (via a glass of wine or chocolate bar) and flush them out successfully. "Clean" also refers to the foods that we eat; fresh and in their natural state, not processed and "lean" means just that—lean and healthy. It doesn't mean a body that's gym-honed to within an inch of its life or one that is scarily skinny. It means a lovely-looking body that's just the right side of athletic... a good mix of curvy, slim, and healthy. But if you want your body to be lean it has to be clean.

CLEAN & LEAN IN A NUTSHELL

The first step to becoming clean and lean is to follow my 14-day Clean & Lean Kickstart plan. This is covered in more detail in Chapter 6, but—in brief—it consists of three meals, plus snacks, a day; you're also allowed one cup of (organic) coffee or tea every day plus up to six cups of (organic) green tea. You should drink at least 2.5 liters of still, filtered water every day and no alcohol or fizzy drinks. I'll also be asking you to do some exercises, which you'll learn more about in Chapter 9.

Why dieting is a waste of time

I've spent years studying nutrition—and observing my clients—and I know this for certain. Sure, you can live on processed low-fat food and diet colas for a little while but your body will be so toxic that you'll find it hard to keep the weight off. I've seen this happen thousands of times. People come to me who have tried every single diet out there, yet they can't stay slim for long. They cut carbs, they count calories, they ban whole food groups, and they spend their lives weighing and measuring out food. But this type of dieting is a complete waste of time; it might help you to drop a dress size or tighten your belt for a while, but you'll gain it back eventually because your body will still be toxic and it's unsustainable—who wants to live like this? And so the cycle of dieting, feeling miserable and deprived, losing and gaining weight continues.

For me there is no "happy" in a steamed chicken breast and a bowl of dust. I want you to enjoy your food and love your life. You can have coffee every day—even during the 14-day Clean & Lean Kickstart. After this time, you can also have a blowout—an eat-whatever-you-like "cheat meal" (see p. 169)—once a week too. Yes, really! All you need to do is follow a few simple rules, which I'll explain in the course of this book, and get into a few habits that will become second nature after a while. You'll quickly become clean, then lean, as your body sheds the fat it's been holding on to for years. And it'll last a lifetime. Imagine that, permanent, beautiful transformation.

*top tip

Remember, it's all about a happy life. There are no crazy rules, no food-measuring, no calorie-counting...

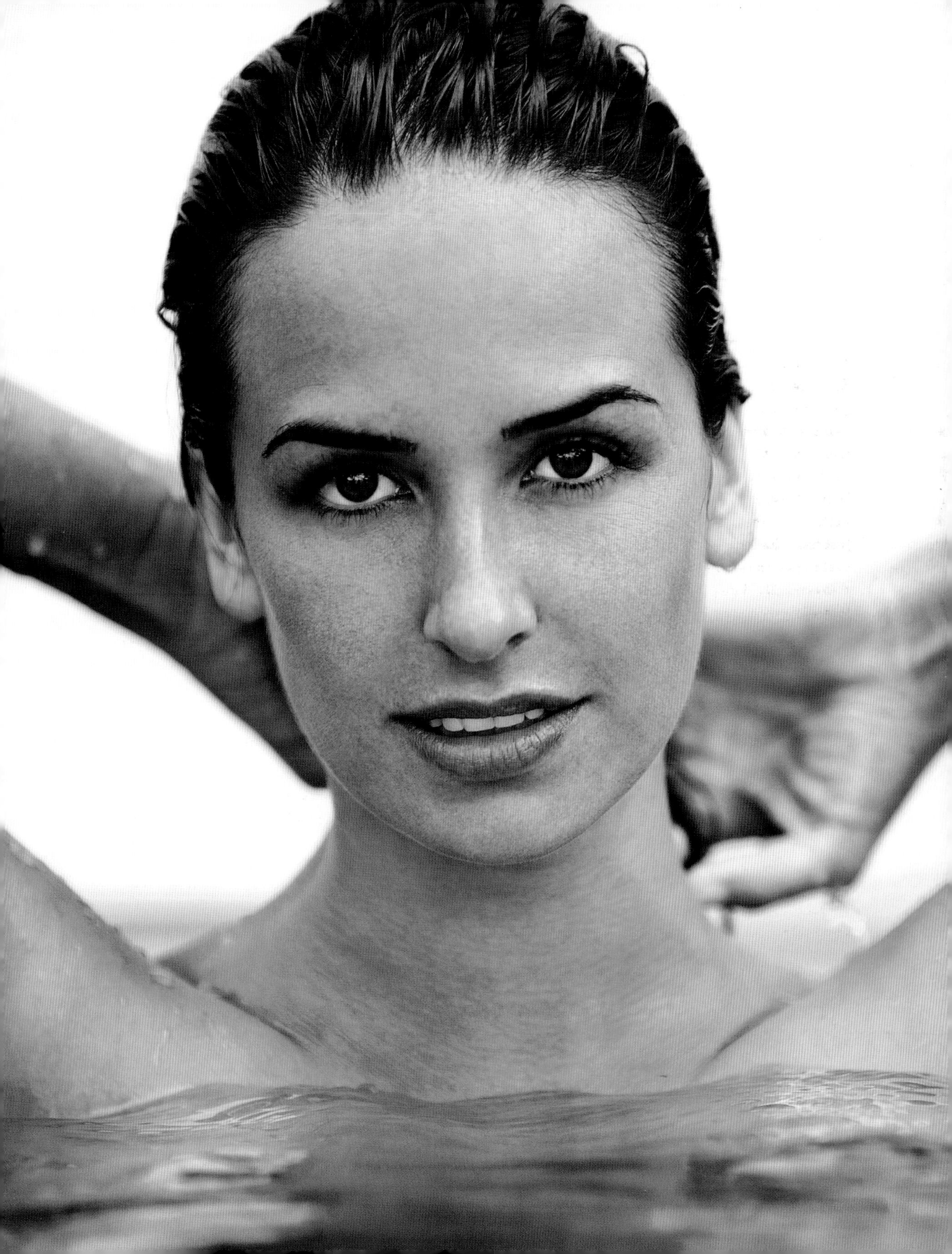

WHY WE EAT THE WAY WE EAT

I love food! Christiane and I start talking about lunch before we finish breakfast, and my happiest moments are when I am eating good food with family and friends. But I also understand that we all have a complicated relationship with food and often our behaviors are driven by things that happened in our childhood—trauma, abuse, self-punishment, and financial hardship, to name a few.

Let me share a little bit of my own story with you now.

I grew up in quite a poor home where sometimes there was no food on the table. Other times, there wasn't even a table. There was, however, lots of love, laughter, and singing and, no matter how bad things were, my dad was a super-hero and always made things OK. So I feel very lucky to have had the things I had, but being hungry sucked. It is an enduring and powerful memory from my childhood and it affected my relationship with food for years without me ever knowing. I never understood why I ate the way I did—why I would binge eat until I felt sick and could hardly move. And, regardless of what I'd already eaten, I could never leave anything on my plate. I guess all this came from a deep belief that food was scarce and that there wasn't enough for me. Now that I understand what was driving this behavior, I can tell the hungry little glutton inside me that there is plenty of food and that I don't need to eat everything I see. Recognizing this has really helped me to deal with it, and I hope this may get some of you thinking about the eating habits you have that aren't working for you and why they might have evolved in the first place.

One of my other enduring memories is of my mother's beautiful cooking. She instilled in me a deep appreciation for good food cooked well.

My mother noticed that whenever I had sugar I would throw a tantrum and run around in circles for twenty minutes, then cry for an hour (that still happens to this day), so my childhood was largely sugar-free, apart from the epic binges I managed at grandparents' and friends' houses. At the time, being the only sugar-free kid didn't feel so good but I'm grateful for it now as I feel it has played a big part in me feeling so healthy as an adult. My relationship with food is now one of unconditional love: I love food and food loves me.

Food is one of our main life sources. It nourishes us, keeps us strong, and can make us look and feel amazing, lifting our mood and our energy levels. When you view it in this way and eat foods that are good for you, the weight will drop off. But when you view food as the enemy, as something that is "bad" for you, you will remain stuck in that all-too-common cycle of deprivation and "reward"—the reward being a binge on fatty, sugary foods that gives you a fleeting high, followed by a feeling of sickness, tiredness and, ultimately, guilt and shame. And then the cycle starts all over again.

I want to help you change your relationship with food and see it as something to be enjoyed while you're relaxed and happy, not something that stirs up feelings of despair. I want you to love food and to find as much joy in it as Christiane and I do.

Why toxins make you fat

Your body stores toxins (poisonous substances produced by living cells or organisms) in your fat cells. If you're dieting simply by not eating (bad idea), your body will slowly lose fat, so that the toxins will have nowhere to go but back into your system, making you feel miserable, deprived, tired all the time and you'll go to bed dreaming of chocolate bars every night. This is why most people feel so rotten within a few days of starting a diet. Your body then quickly decides it doesn't like feeling this way, so it holds on to fat in order to store the toxins.

A toxic body will find it difficult to digest or retain nutrients properly. And a high-calorie diet may not be high in vitamins and minerals and so that's often why overweight people are so hungry—they're hungry for nutrients. So clean toxins out of your system and you'll find losing weight is simple. To become truly Clean, you need to clear out your excretory system, which is responsible for removing toxic waste from your body. So if you want a Lean, lovely body you need this system to be clean and functioning as best it can. The excretory system is made up of the three main detoxers—your skin (through sweating), your liver, and your kidneys.

I've cleaned out people's diets in the past and the weight loss has been dramatic. And we're not talking about crash diets or starvation—these people were eating three meals a day, plus coffee and snacks, and they still lost weight effortlessly and quickly. How did they do it? They removed toxins from their diet and they got clean.

What else makes you toxic?

We all come into daily contact with toxins. Fumes from cars, dirt in the air, toxins in cleaning products, tap water—you name it, it's toxic. But let's face it, we'd lead a pretty weird life if we tried to avoid these things altogether. Several people also argue that our bodies are perfectly capable of dealing with toxins—and they're right, up to a point. Unfortunately, however, we're exposed to so many of them nowadays—especially in food and drink—that we've become overloaded. So it makes sense to limit our bodies' exposure to toxins in the first place.

Tap water, in my opinion, is best avoided. A 2008 inquiry by the Associated Press found traces of prescription and over-the-counter medication in drinking water supplies across the USA. These traces were incredibly small, so there's no need to panic, but it makes sense to make sure that everything you eat and drink is as clean as possible, so buy a water filter pitcher and keep it in your fridge.

Are some toxins worse than others?

Absolutely. For example, caffeine is better for us than alcohol. In moderation and when drunk properly (see Chapter 3 for more information on this), coffee can actually burn fat, give you a great hit of antioxidants, and improve your performance in the gym. It's only when you have too much of it that it becomes fattening because it places stress on the adrenal glands, disturbs sleep, dehydrates you, and may stop you drinking enough water. However, if you drink good-quality, organic, black coffee with a splash of organic milk, one cup a day can be a good thing.

Alcohol, on the other hand, has few if any benefits. There is some evidence that red wine is an antioxidant and can boost heart health but otherwise alcohol is toxic and causes damage to almost every part of the body, from the internal organs, to the skin and the waistline.

After 14 days, can I reintroduce toxins?

By the time you've read this book, I promise you won't view foods like cake and chocolate in the same way. I appreciate you may still want them occasionally but the Clean & Lean plan allows for that. So to answer the question: during the 14-day Clean & Lean Kickstart, you can have a cup of (organic) tea or coffee every day. After this, you can have up to two cups a day. You're not allowed any alcohol during the 14-day kickstart and, ideally, I'd like you to avoid it for a further four weeks after that. However, if you absolutely must have it, only drink once a week for four weeks and then have only red wine or clear spirits (Grey Goose vodka is the least processed one). After that, you can drink in moderation (I'll explain how to make healthy choices in Chapter 3). Cutting back on alcohol will give you such speedy weight loss that I promise you it will be worth it.

CLEAN & LEAN FUNDAMENTALS

* Your past does not equal your future
* Be kind to yourself: let go of shame and guilt and accept who you are
* Be kind to the planet—it's good for you, I promise! Eat fresh, organic, and local
* Move your body every day, your body loves to move
* The word diet literally means "the foods you eat." It's something that you do forever, not just for 2 weeks at a time
* Any transformation that happens in your body happens in your mind first
* Beautiful is how you feel not how you look
* Stay Clean & Lean forever!

WHERE ARE TOXINS FOUND?

These are the most fattening toxins:

* Sugar
* Alcohol
* Soft drinks
* Processed foods
* Processed "diet" foods
* Excess caffeine
* Cortisol—the stress hormone

*top tip

If it couldn't swim, fly or run or it didn't grow off the land—don't eat it!

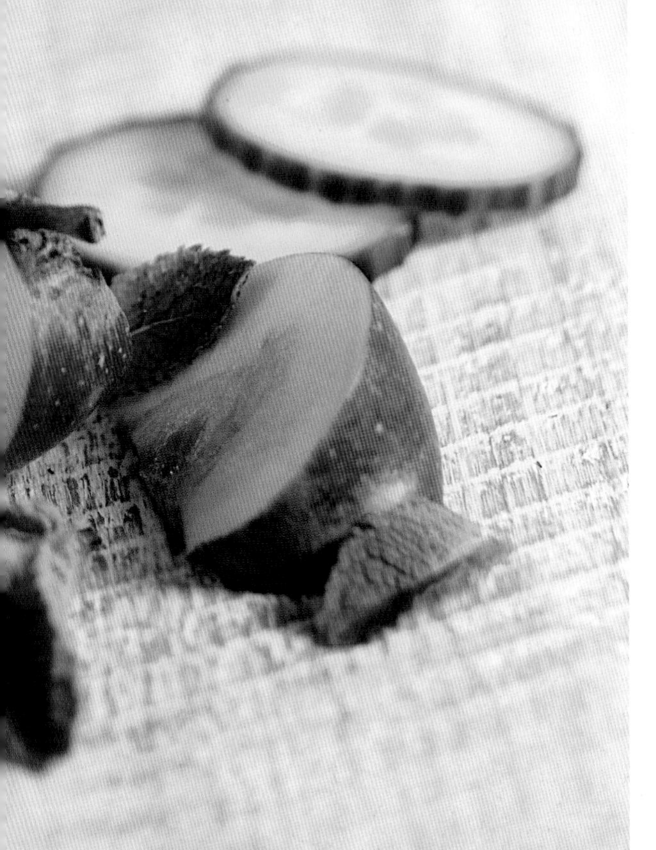

What makes foods clean?

Clean foods are those that:

* haven't changed much from their natural state—for example, an apple in a bowl still resembles the apple on the tree, whereas a potato chip (having been heavily processed) looks nothing like a potato
* don't need any added artificial flavor
* don't last for months and months; they go bad in the fridge or cupboard after a short while
* generally contain fewer than five or six ingredients
* have no ingredients that you can't pronounce or recognize
* don't list sugar as their main ingredient (or as one of the first three)
* don't make you feel bloated, gassy, or uncomfortably full
* satisfy you, so that you're not hungry after eating them.

ANTIOXIDANTS

I'll be talking about antioxidants a lot in this book. Antioxidants are substances that protect your cells from the harmful effects of free radicals (found in the environment, chemicals, rays from the sun, and tobacco smoke). These free radicals damage your cells and basically age you—from your skin to your heart. Antioxidants mop up free radicals and slow down the aging (and therefore degenerative) process. They are mostly found in brightly colored fruits and vegetables, especially those with high levels of vitamin A, C, and E. Lycopene is a particularly powerful health-boosting antioxidant that gives tomatoes their red color.

Antioxidant-rich foods include:

* tomatoes (they're packed with lycopene)
* dark red, blue, or black fruits with thin skin (blueberries, blackberries, strawberries, etc.)
* sweet potatoes
* red, green, yellow, and orange bell peppers
* avocados
* dark greens (spinach, arugula, etc.)
* Clean & Lean Beauty Food and Berry Burn (bodyism.com)

Why organic food helps keep you slim

Eating good-quality food that's organic is investing in your health. I often hear people say that it's too expensive to eat organic, and my response is to do the best job you can do with what you can afford and remember that investing in your health now is what leads to a happy, healthy, and long life. You might also save on medical bills in the long run.

Organic food is likely to contain fewer toxins (such as pesticides) and other additives found in non-organic food (such as aspartame, tartrazine, MSG, and hydrogenated fats). Farming methods today are very often driven by profit: pesticides are sprayed on crops to keep the produce alive and untouched by insects for as long as possible (for example, the longer a strawberry stays fresh, the more it's likely to sell, keeping profits higher for the farmers and the food manufacturers). Similarly, non-organic animals are fed more cheaply (and with more toxins) than organic ones. A 2012 study from the University of Stirling even found that current pesticide use has led to a decline in bee colonies.

In my humble opinion, organic foods also contain more health-boosting minerals and vitamins, higher levels of vitamin C, calcium, magnesium, iron, antioxidants, and omega-3 fatty acids—all of which can help to make you healthier, stronger, and slimmer. Take organic milk, for example, which contains up to 68 percent more omega-3 essential fatty acids than regular milk, helping your body to burn fat around your waist (more on this in Chapter 5). There was a study a few years ago that suggested there was no difference between organic food and sprayed food. However, it just makes sense to me that the less pesticides and hormones your food has in it, the better it is for you. If you don't agree, that's fine!

Genetically modified (GM) crops and ingredients are also banned under organic standards. However, GM crops are also fed to non-organic livestock, which ends up as non-organic pork, bacon, milk, cheese, and other dairy products found in our supermarkets. So always, always pick organic food, wherever possible—especially when it comes to meat, dairy, and eggs. And try to stay away from GM food. Again, you do what you can with what you've got. If you can't get or afford organic then just get as fresh as possible and wash your vegetables thoroughly.

To give you a clearer picture, here's my "Bad, Better and Best" guide to buying organic:

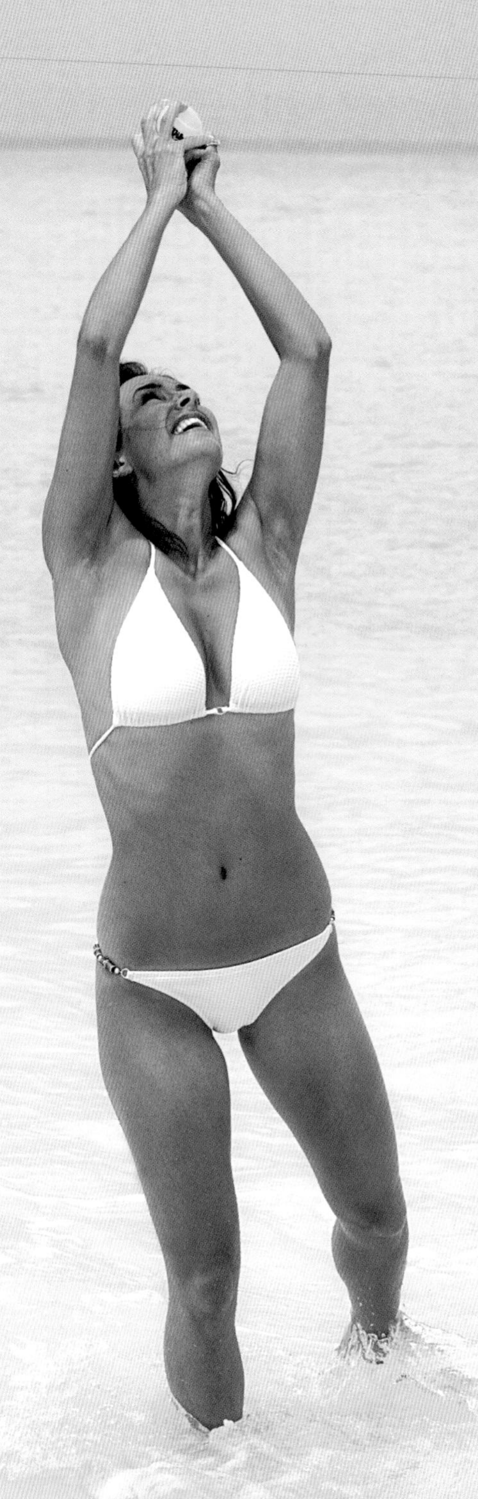

BAD	BETTER	BEST
Cage-bred chicken—raised on grains and antibiotics	**Free-range chicken breasts**—contain more omega-3 and omega-6 than conventionally raised chicken	**Organic chicken breasts**—contain more protein, more polyunsaturated fat (the good kind) and less saturated fat (the bad kind)
Battery caged eggs—lower in omega-3's	**Free-range eggs**	**Organic free-range eggs**—more fat-burning, health-boosting omega 3-s, and they taste better too
Margarine—usually full of chemicals and heavily processed	**Butter**—a more natural option, but some brands still contain additives	**Organic butter**—natural and free of preservatives and additives
Instant coffee—coffee is one of the most sprayed plants in the world, plus processing it into an "instant" form further depletes it of nutrients	**Espresso**—less processed than instant coffee; no milk, sugar or other additives	**Organic espresso with organic cream**—pesticide- and herbicide-free (the cream slows the digestion of the caffeine)
Strawberry yogurt (all the overripe fruit is put into yogurt, meaning more sugar and fewer nutrients), and they even add sugar to these products, especially the low-fat ones	**Strawberries**—500 lbs of pesticide per acre is sprayed on non-organic strawberries—yuck!	**Organic strawberries**—remember—the thinner the skin, the more pesticides are absorbed into the fruit; this is why you should always choose organic for berries and cherries
Supermarket steaks—supermarkets buy cheaply in bulk and often from overseas, which means a longer time from the farm to your table	**Steaks bought from a butcher** (these steaks are usually from locally reared animals)	**Organic steaks**—free from hormones, antibiotics, and nitrates
Cow's milk—contains lactose that can cause digestive issues	**Goat milk**—easier to digest than cow's milk	**Organic rice milk or oat milk**—no cholesterol or saturated fat
Iceberg lettuce—basically green water with almost no nutrients; the lettuce of today has one twentieth of the nutrients it had fifty years ago, due to severely mineral-depleted soil	**Spinach**—very high in magnesium, calcium, antioxidants, and chlorophyll, which cleanses your blood and helps detox your liver	**Organic spinach**—as with non-organic, but with lots more nutrients
Dried fruit—the drying process can lead to significant loss of nutrients	**Fresh fruit**—a delicious source of fiber, vitamins, and minerals	**Organic fruit**—free from toxins
Waxed apples—the really shiny apples look better, but the wax actually drags nutrients from them	**Loose apples in a bag**—a low-GI fruit that is packed with nutrients	**Organic apples**—they may not look as pretty, but they don't contain any nasty toxins, either

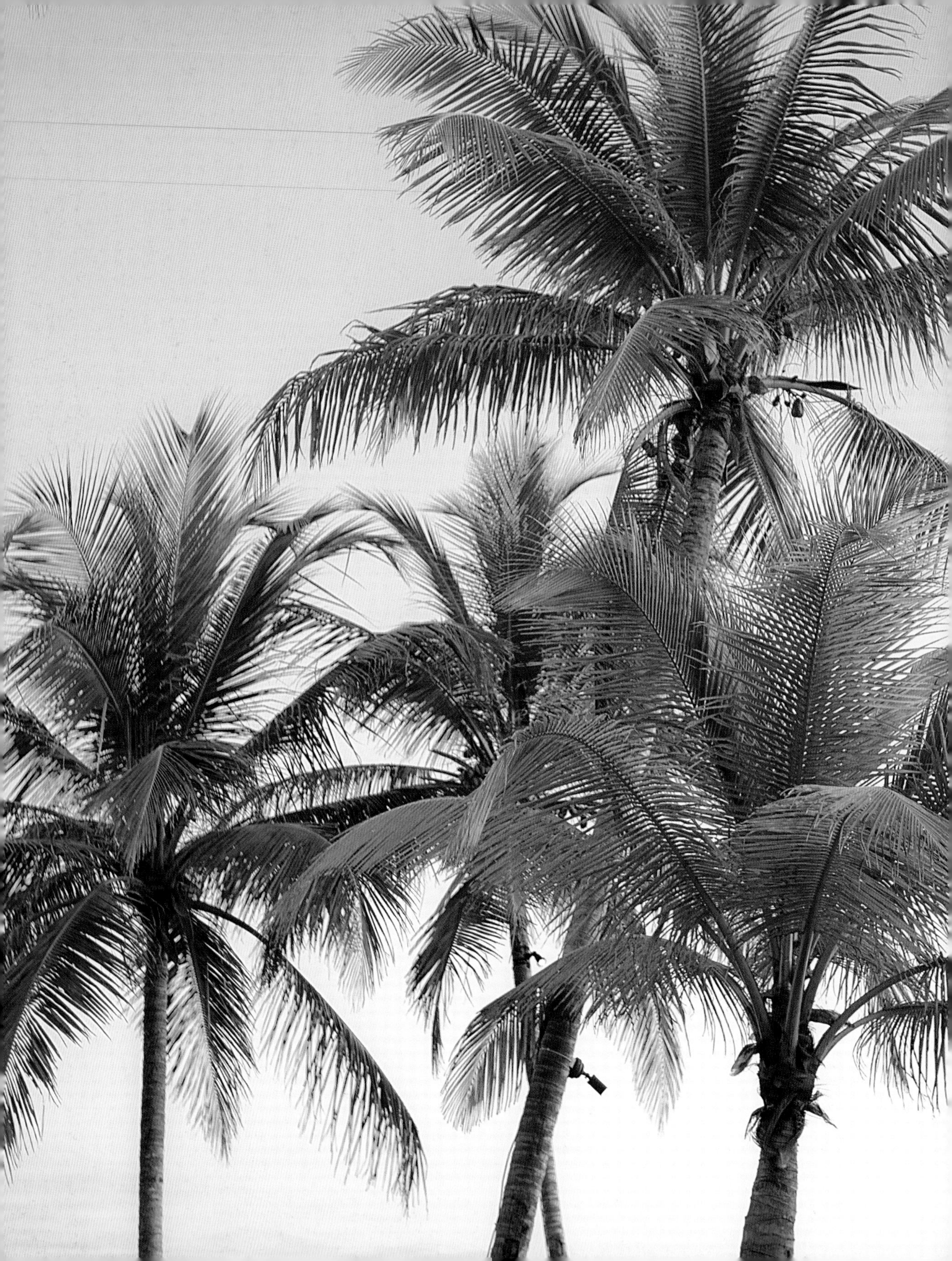

CHAPTER 2

WHY SUGAR IS NOT SO SWEET

THIS CHAPTER WILL REVEAL…

WHY SUGAR IS ADDICTIVE

WHY SUGAR IS SO BAD FOR YOU

HOW TO GIVE SUGAR UP

MOST OF US LOVE SUGAR...

I know I did. And with more than 115 million tons of it produced worldwide each year, it seems I'm not the only one with a sweet tooth. So why do we love it so much?

Sugar—not so sweet

Sugar is perfectly designed to hook us in. It comes to us in the form of pretty pink cupcakes, fluffy marshmallows, light sponge cakes with jam in the middle and creamy chocolate. In fact, just about everything sugary looks and smells delicious. I was watching my baby cousin at his first birthday party the other day, when he got his first hit of sugar from his birthday cake. You could see his little face light up; he loved that sugar and he just wanted more. It was almost scary.

But, in reality, there's nothing to love about refined sugar. It makes us put on weight, increases the size of our liver (a bad thing), makes us unwell, and ages us inside and out, leaving us tired, fat, and wrinkled. As well as being highly addictive, refined sugar drags valuable nutrients out of our body, and it's the number-one reason why, for the first time in history, the children of this generation are predicted to die younger than their parents. This is happening because sugar is a big business with a massive marketing campaign behind it, so it's able to target us from a very early age, making addicts of us all.

Why sugar is physically addictive

Sugar has a similar effect on the brain to pain-killing drugs like morphine and other opiates (such as heroin). These types of drugs produce an almost instant feeling of pleasure, calm, and satisfaction, making them incredibly addictive. When the food manufacturers figured this out, they began producing foods full of sugar. Back in the 1950s, sugar would mainly be found in homemade cakes, but now it's pumped into almost all processed foods, alcoholic and soft drinks, and even so-called "healthy" foods (such as breakfast cereals) and foods aimed at children.

Many of us turn to something sugary for "energy"—and technically, it is a form of energy. But it's a bad type. So yes, you will get a quick burst after eating a chocolate bar, but about ten minutes after that you'll feel even more tired than you were before. That's because sugar quickly hits the bloodstream, creating a rapid rise in blood sugar (a "spike"). But, just as quickly, you then crash (due to insulin being produced from the pancreas), leaving you exhausted. A far better way of getting energy is to eat complex carbohydrates (low-GI fruits, berries), Clean & Lean proteins, vegetables, drink plenty of water, and exercise regularly. If you do all these things, you won't need to rely on something as toxic as sugar to keep you energized.

Studies also suggest that the ability to tell between sweet and bitter is hardwired into our DNA. It helped us to survive in cavemen times when we needed to know the difference between what was poisonous and what was safe to eat. We are also one of the only animals that cannot produce our own vitamin C—we need to get it from what we consume. And vitamin C is found mostly in things that are sweet. So it's reasonable to assume that we're hardwired to want food that is sweet and probably abundant in vitamin C (most vitamin-C rich fruits likes berries and oranges are very sweet). This wasn't so much of a problem in the days when we had to hunt and gather our own food—cupcakes don't grow on trees. These days, however, they're everywhere and sugar is far more available and comes in far worse forms. After all, the natural sugar found in fruit is one thing but the processed rubbish found in candy and cakes is something else altogether.

*top tip

Avoid overripe fruits. The riper a fruit is the more sugar it contains, meaning the higher your chance of storing that sugar as fat. So the next time you're choosing which piece of fruit to eat, don't go for the softest because it contains the most sugar.

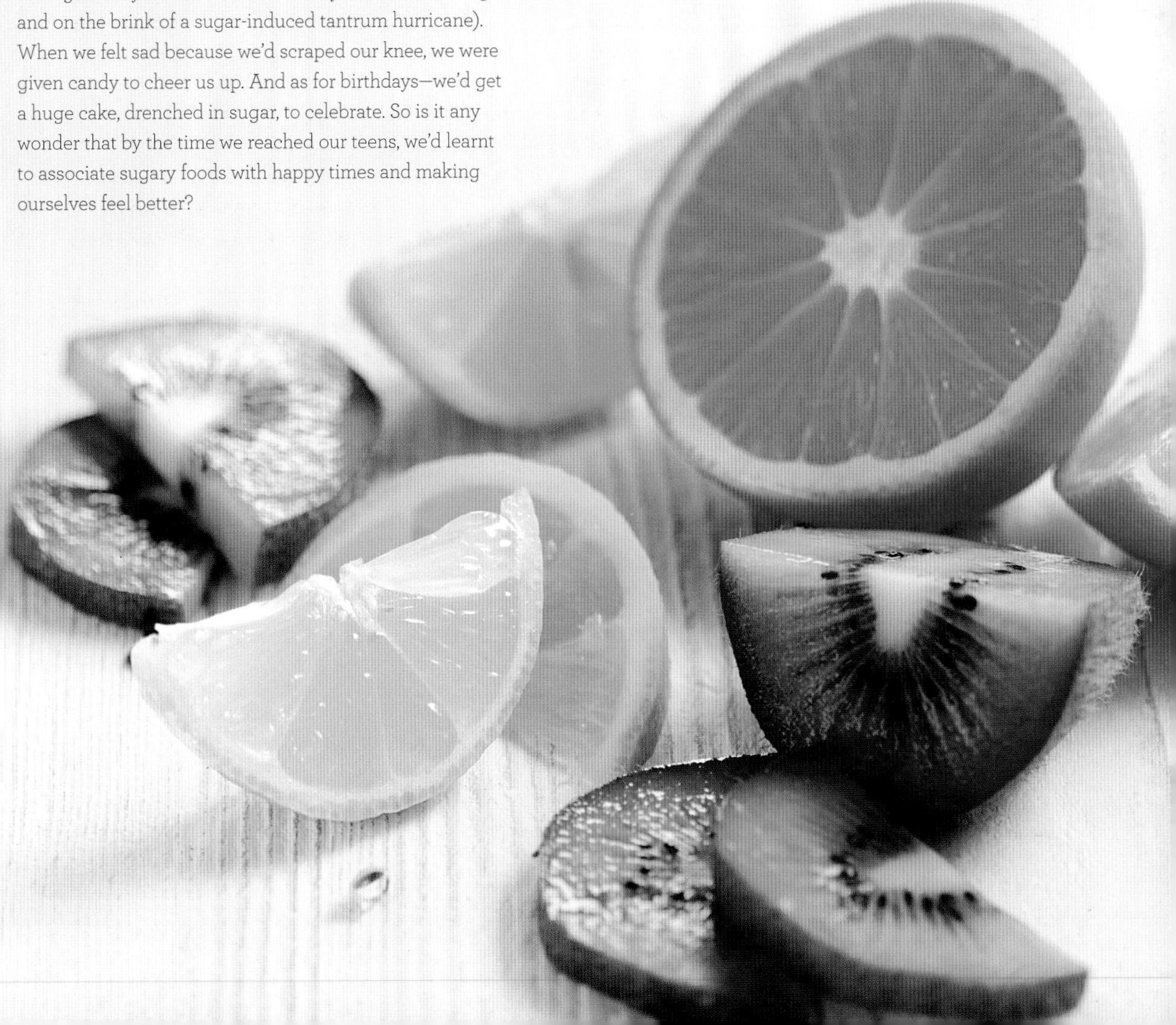

Why sugar is emotionally addictive

For most of us, when we were growing up, sugary foods were used as a "reward" by our parents, grandparents, and almost everybody else we knew as children. If we got good grades at school, we'd be given sweets on the way home, to say, "Well done." When we stayed with our grandparents and behaved ourselves, we got cake (actually I got cake at my grandparents' house, no matter what I did; I think it was their way of thanking my dad for being such a cheeky teenager—they'd send me home red-eyed and screaming and on the brink of a sugar-induced tantrum hurricane). When we felt sad because we'd scraped our knee, we were given candy to cheer us up. And as for birthdays—we'd get a huge cake, drenched in sugar, to celebrate. So is it any wonder that by the time we reached our teens, we'd learnt to associate sugary foods with happy times and making ourselves feel better?

I had a client once who was hopelessly addicted to sugar. When she first came to see me, her diet was appalling. She had to eat something sugary every day, especially after meals or whenever she was stressed or sad. When I dug a little deeper, it turned out that her mother was seriously ill when she was very young and her father had to take care of her a lot when her mother was in and out of the hospital. As a toddler, if she was upset or had trouble sleeping, her father would dip her pacifier in some honey to soothe her. As a result, she always turned to sugar for comfort. The association she had between sugar and love was really deep and strong.

Many of us do exactly the same thing as this client: when we're heartbroken, lonely, sad, or stressed we turn to sugar to make us feel better, gorging on ice cream, cake, or chocolate to cheer ourselves up. But guess what? Sugary foods don't cheer us up. They make us fat, stressed, old-looking, and ill. So the next time you go to eat something sugary because you've been dumped or you've had a bad day at work, stop and ask yourself: "Will this make my problems better or worse?" Look past the pretty pink icing and see sugar for the fattening toxin that it is.

MARIES' STORY

"I used to be a huge sugar addict. I saw a chocolate bar in the afternoon as a break from work. I also loved a cupcake or some shortbread with my latte and some cookies with a hot cup of tea. But James made me realize that it wasn't the sugar I was enjoying, but the things I associated it with. In fact, when I thought about it, I felt worse after eating it. It made my stomach bloat and my energy levels plummet. When I stopped eating it, I felt lighter, slimmer, and my skin glowed. Now I rarely touch the stuff, and I don't miss it at all."

Why sugar is so bad for you

Over the last fifty years, the Western world has doubled its consumption of processed sugar (the type found in cookies, soft drinks, and ice cream, for example) and, during this time, rates of obesity and heart disease have soared. Of course, sugar isn't solely responsible—but it is largely to blame. If you think I'm being overly dramatic about it, Google "Harmful effects of processed sugar" and you'll get about six million links. Millions of people (especially in America and the UK, where processed sugar consumption is highest) are fat, unwell, and living uncomfortably, getting by on all sorts of medications just to keep their overloaded bodies going.

In the autumn of 2009, the American Heart Association (AHA) released a statement urging people to cut back on processed sugar. They advised that women should have no more than six teaspoons a day, which is around 100 calories' worth (and remember, this is the absolute most you should be having—ideally you shouldn't really have any processed sugar at all, unless it comes from natural sources like fruit), yet the average American has 22 teaspoons a day! To give you an idea, just one can of diet drink contains around eight teaspoons of sugar; imagine how much sugar you're eating if you add cookies, cakes, candy, and everything else sugary on top of that.

In the last 20 years, sugar consumption in the US has increased from 25 lbs to 135 lbs per person per year! At the turn of the 19th century (1887–90), the average consumption was only 5 lbs per person per year.

What eating sugar can do to you

Sugar makes you fat: your body cannot process too much of it, so it gets stored as fat. Plus it also makes fat-burning even harder—if you're eating sugar every day, all the gym sessions in the world won't shift that excess flab.

As we've seen (see p. 24), sugar is also addictive, so once you start eating it, it's very hard to stop. This is why you very rarely find a packet of half-finished cookies. Stop the cycle by not starting it. Find comfort in other things—have a camomile or a green tea or some blueberries with yogurt and nuts with cinnamon (perfect!). Go for a brisk walk, have a long bath, paint your nails, phone a friend—anything to distract your mind from having more sugar.

Sugar leaches your body of vitamin B: any mental, physical or emotional stress drains vitamin B from your body—as does sugar—which causes exhaustion. If you add sugar on to the end of a stressed-out day, you're getting a double whammy of vitamin B depletion. Vitamin B keeps your metabolism healthy, boosts your energy levels, keeps skin, hair and nails healthy, and keeps your immunity strong.

Burning body fat has a lot to do with controlling your insulin levels. But sugar spikes raise your insulin levels, leading to faster fat storage and this is the real reason why so many of us in the Western world are either overweight or obese. Sugar, not fat, is making us fatter. In a healthy, slim person, 40 percent of the sugar they eat is converted straight to fat; in an overweight person, up to 60 percent is converted straight to fat and stored right around their hips, stomach, and thighs. Think about it: up to 60 percent of that cupcake is heading straight for your tummy, hips, and thighs, where it will remain for a very long time.

Sugar lowers energy levels: processed sugar causes a huge and damaging increase in your blood-sugar levels, giving you a quick burst of energy, which is soon followed by a long, hard crash, leaving you tired, hungry and, eventually, fat.

Sugar wears out your organs: it forces your internal organs to cope with changes in your body chemistry which means that your kidneys and pancreas can become worn out long before you stop needing them. Hence the increase in late-onset diabetes.

Too much sugar depletes vitamin and mineral stores in the body, which may impact on the immune system. So you become ill more frequently and for longer.

It's time to get real and remember that sugar is a nuclear fat bomb exploding all over your body. If you eat it every day, you'll always struggle to lose weight and you'll never have a flat tummy.

The worst offenders

White refined sugar—the stuff you get in packages and stir into your tea or cake mixtures.

Fruit juices—most commercial fruit juice is basically sugared water with all the fiber extracted and very little vitamin and mineral content. It is best either to have a small glass of freshly squeezed juice or, better still, a piece of whole fruit.

Bad carbs—white, non-organic pasta, bread, cereals, and cereal bars are the worst offenders. Even seemingly healthy brown carbs (like whole wheat bread) contain sugar.

Alcohol—it's literally all sugar.

Cakes, candy, cookies, ice cream—need I say more?

So-called "low-fat foods"—such as diet yogurts, most breakfast cereals (more on these in Chapter 3), health bars, muffins, and energy drinks, are all packed with sugar to give them flavor. A common trick of the food manufacturer is to label a food as being "low fat" when there was no fat in there to begin with. This is most common with breakfast cereals (again, see more on why you should never eat these in Chapter 3).

Any ingredient ending in "ose"—sugar is often hidden in words ending with "ose" (sucrose, maltose, lactose, dextrose, and fructose, for example). Another common name is "syrup," the very worst being "high-fructose corn syrup" (HFCS)—one of the cheapest sweeteners around, it boosts fat-storing hormones, while a recent study at the University of Pennsylvania found that it also increases the hunger hormone; it's found in sweets, cereal bars, fruit drinks, ketchup, mayonnaise, pasta sauce, and even salad dressing, so always read the labels.

Anything that lists sugar—in any of its guises—in the first three ingredients.

You basically need to steer clear of any sweeteners, especially the artificial ones which are made of toxic chemicals. Remember that most packaged foods contain sweeteners along with other additives that you really want to avoid if you want a slim waist. Learn to read labels and avoid anything fake or toxic looking.

As a rough guide, here are some of the things you should be looking out for:

- high-fructose corn syrup
- white sugar
- brown sugar
- cane sugar
- sucrose
- dextrose
- fructose
- sucanat
- turbinado sugar
- beet sugar
- maltose
- sorbitol
- mannitol
- erythritol
- aspartame
- saccharin
- Nutrisweet
- Splenda
- cylcamate
- sucralose
- Acesulfame-K

If you are having a real tough time quitting the habit and you need a little sweetness just to get through the day, I would recommend stevia. It's a herb that's 200 times sweeter than sugar. Another natural source of sweetness is xylitol, which you can buy in granulated form (so it's good for adding to hot drinks) and it releases energy slowly.

SUGAR IN FRUIT

The best form of sugar is raw fruit. So the next time you have a sweet craving, eat some in-season thin-skinned fruit, such as berries, apples, pears, cherries, or green grapes. Always make sure you eat these with protein and/or fat to slow down the speed at which the sugar hits your bloodstream.

Having said that, fruit—though packed with goodness—is still high in sugar, so don't eat too much of it. Yes, we all need "five a day" (i.e. five portions of fruit and vegetables a day), but the majority of this should come from vegetables. Go easy on fruit for a few weeks, and you'll be amazed at the difference it makes to your waistline, energy levels, and how much (or how little) you bloat. Berries are the best fruit of all, so eat more of those than any other fruit.

WHAT ABOUT HONEY?

Raw honey, pure maple syrup, brown rice syrup, molasses (which are packed full of calcium, iron, B vitamins, and potassium), manuka honey (which is full of antioxidants), barley malt, stevia, xylotol, and agave are all OK in moderation. But the key word here is "moderation." Like fruit, these things have their benefits—and they're certainly better for you than the processed sugar you find in candy—but they should still only form a small part of your diet.

*top tip

The darker the fruit, the better. Dark fruits tend to have very thin skin, so they need to produce more antioxidants to protect themselves from the sun.

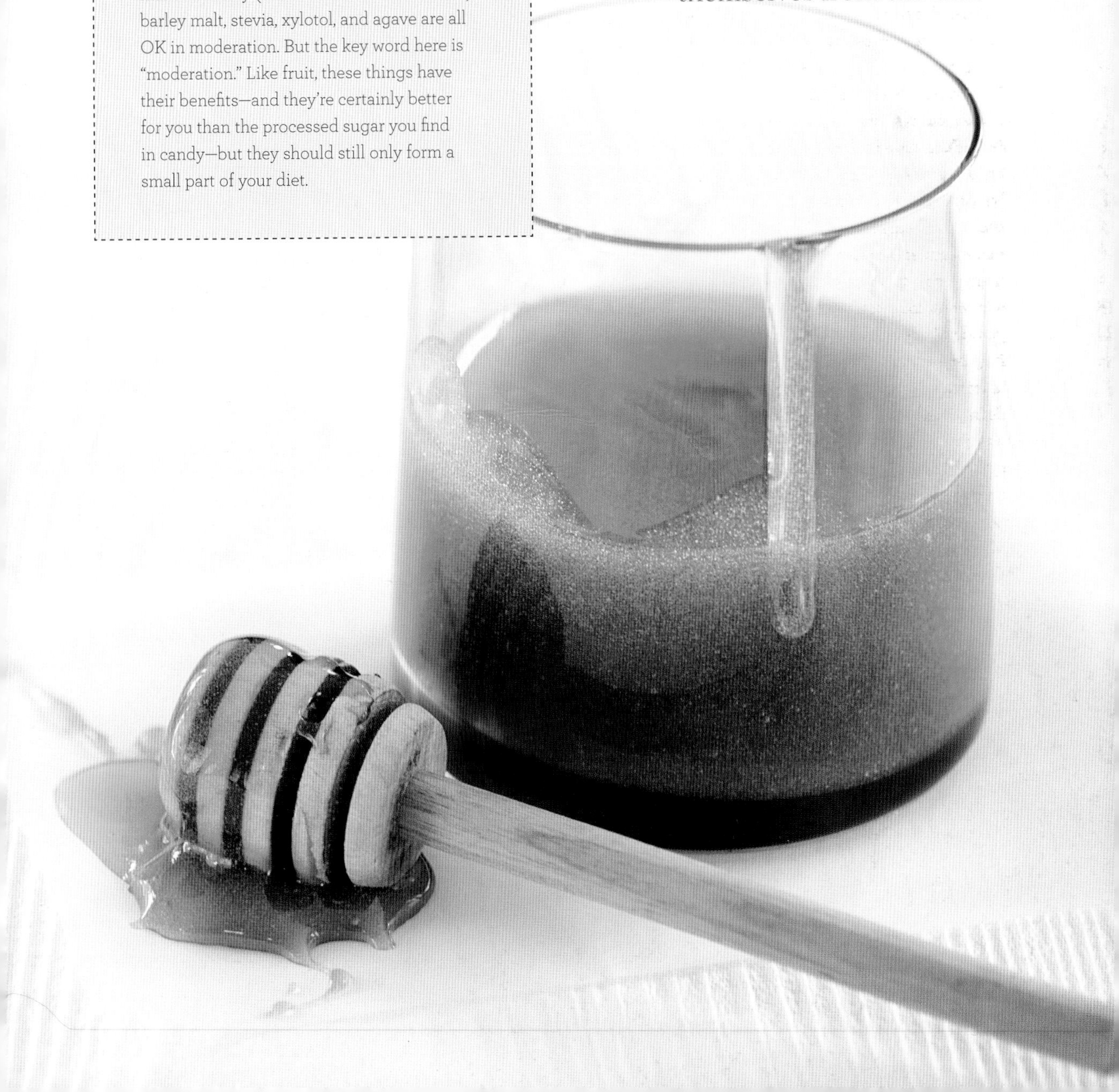

HOW TO GIVE UP SUGAR

You really need to give sugar up if you want to be Clean & Lean. All the other things we're going to talk about in this book—like coffee—can be reintroduced once you've completed the 14-day Clean & Lean Kickstart. But sugar? It's so nasty, so toxic, and so utterly bad for you that it's better to just ditch it altogether. And here's how:

Don't ever use sugar as a reward

Ask yourself this—how is giving yourself early wrinkles, a bloated stomach and fat around your middle a "reward?" See sugar for what it is—a nasty toxin that's dyed a pretty color to lure you in, and which then makes you fat and unwell. Reward yourself with something else instead, like a beauty treatment or a new book.

Eat plenty of chromium

Chromium helps to control your blood-sugar levels and banish sugar cravings. Good sources include eggs, molasses, liver, kidney, wholegrains, nuts, mushrooms, and asparagus. It should not be eaten in large quantities if you are diabetic.

Supplement your diet with glutamine

Glutamine is an amino acid that squashes sugar cravings. It can be found in most health-food shops; take one tablespoon in a small glass of water whenever you get a sugar craving.

Include dark meat proteins in your diet

Sugar cravings often come from a lack of protein in your diet. Try eating darker meats, such as chicken legs, beef and lamb. Dark meats contain more purines, which have more satisfying nutrients than lighter meats, like chicken breasts or fish, so will help to prevent sugar cravings. In fact, if you're having a sugar craving, try having a slice of chicken or some nuts to banish the urge for sugar.

Take Bodyism supplements

Bodyism Body Brilliance supplements are packed with super greens, chromium plus cinnamon, which helps regulate your blood-sugar levels, boosting energy levels in turn and reducing sugar cravings throughout the day. Bodyism fish oil Omega Brilliance contains essential fatty acids, which are important for optimal health and can help reduce cravings for sugar, as your body is full of good fats.

Bodyism products are available at bodyism.com.

How to eat sugar

If you feel you absolutely must have sugar, there are some rules you should stick to that will help with damage limitation:

1 Always eat sugar at the end of a meal (never before). By eating your protein first (remember—you must eat some protein with every meal), you leave less room for cravings, plus this prevents blood-sugar peaks and crashes.

2 Eat good sugar—as good as possible. That means raw, in-season, thin-skinned fruits or some really good-quality honey—though not too much. Once you start cutting back on sugar, you'll be amazed at how quickly you lose the taste for it, and when you do have some you'll need a lot less than you did before.

3 Never, ever eat sugar on its own (and this includes fruit and honey)—always eat with some protein and "good fat" (try a handful of nuts or natural yogurt). This is because protein and fat slow the rate at which sugar floods into your bloodstream and if sugar hits your bloodstream quickly—as it would after a huge cupcake, for example—you'll feel quickly high, then very quickly low. The slower it hits your blood, the less of a rush you'll get, which means less of a slump.

***it's easy**

All the advice in this book is easy to follow and will leave you looking and feeling strong and healthy.

Overleaf is my "Bad, Better, and Best" guide on how to clean out bad, processed sugars from your diet and replace them with less toxic ones, once you've completed the 14-day Clean & Lean Kickstart (see Chapter 6). If you fancy something in the "Bad" column, pick the one in the "Better" column instead. Or, for a body like Elle's, go for the one in the "Best" column!

BAD	BETTER	BEST
White sugar—your body can't process much sugar, so the rest gets stored as fat. It also depletes your body's vitamin and mineral stores and leaves you feeling exhausted	**Brown sugar**—contains molasses, which provide some minerals such as calcium, iron, and magnesium	**Manuka honey**—full of antioxidants, so a much better way to satisfy your sweet tooth, but only in moderation
Chocolate-coated cookies—full of sugar, wheat, and gluten which can cause inflammation	**Dark chocolate**—a tasty source of antioxidants	**Organic dark chocolate**—the darker the chocolate the better
Candy—nothing but sugar and preservatives	**Dried fruit**—natural sugars rather than highly processed sugar	**Whole piece of fruit plus a handful of almonds**—again, protein with sugar helps prevent a sugar crash
Breakfast cereal—generally high in sugar and low in nutrients and keeps your body craving more sugar	**Wheat-free (oat-based) muesli**—oats are a slow-release source of carbohydrate with lots of fiber	**Super Breakfast** (see p. 87)
Canned fruit salad—high in sodium that can cause water retention	**Thick-skinned fruit salad** (bananas, oranges, and watermelon) —fresh fruit contains vital vitamins and minerals, but you lose some of these by peeling off the skin	**Thin-skinned fruit salad with mixed seeds**—thin, dark-skinned fruits are antioxidant-rich and, as you eat the skin, you don't lose any of the benefits
Low-fat yogurt—generally higher in sugar and with fewer nutrients than the full-fat option	**Organic, full-fat yogurt**—rich in conjugated linoleic acid (CLA) that helps burn body fat	**Organic kefir**—a fermented milk that is super-rich in probiotics, which help improve digestion
Ice pop—purely sugar and chemicals	**Fruit juice**—refreshing, a good vitamin fix, but a lot of sugar, too	**Fresh, organic fruit**—less sugar and rich in fiber to help regulate blood sugar levels
Shop-bought cake—packed with sugar and full of preservatives to prolong its shelf-life	**Fresh cake from a bakery**—still unhealthy, but at least it will be fresh and made with fresh ingredients	**Homemade cake**—made with fruit as the sweetener and no white sugar—a much cleaner way to enjoy a treat

BAD	BETTER	BEST
Cookies—full of salt, sugar, and unhealthy fats	**Oatcakes with peanut butter**—the oatcakes keep you full and the peanut butter provides essential protein	**Rice cakes with organic nut butter**—the perfect blend of proteins, carbohydrates, and healthy fats
Ice cream—milk held together with tons of sugar; most people can't digest dairy properly and this lowers your ability to burn fat	**Organic ice cream**—contains fewer toxins and is free from hormones and antibiotics	**Natural, full-fat organic yogurt with pecans**—contains a lot less sugar and the fat and protein helps fill you up
Muesli/granola bar—stuck together with sugar; don't be fooled by their healthy image	**Homemade flaked granola**—less sugar, fewer preservatives and made with Clean & Lean ingredients	**Oatmeal with organic nuts and seeds**—low-GI, full of fiber and omega 3's
Milk chocolate bar or packet of sweets—this is a convenient pocket-sized fat bomb	**Dark chocolate**—less sugar and has a higher antioxidant content	**Organic dark chocolate with hazelnuts**—fewer toxins and contains healthy fat and fiber to help keep you feeling full
Croissant—zero fiber and soaked in bad fats; probably the worst breakfast ever unless you have a donut with a cigarette—that's the worst!	**Muffin from a health-food shop**—contains more fiber but is still full of sugar and wheat	**Homemade muffin made with Clean & Lean ingredients**—rich in fiber

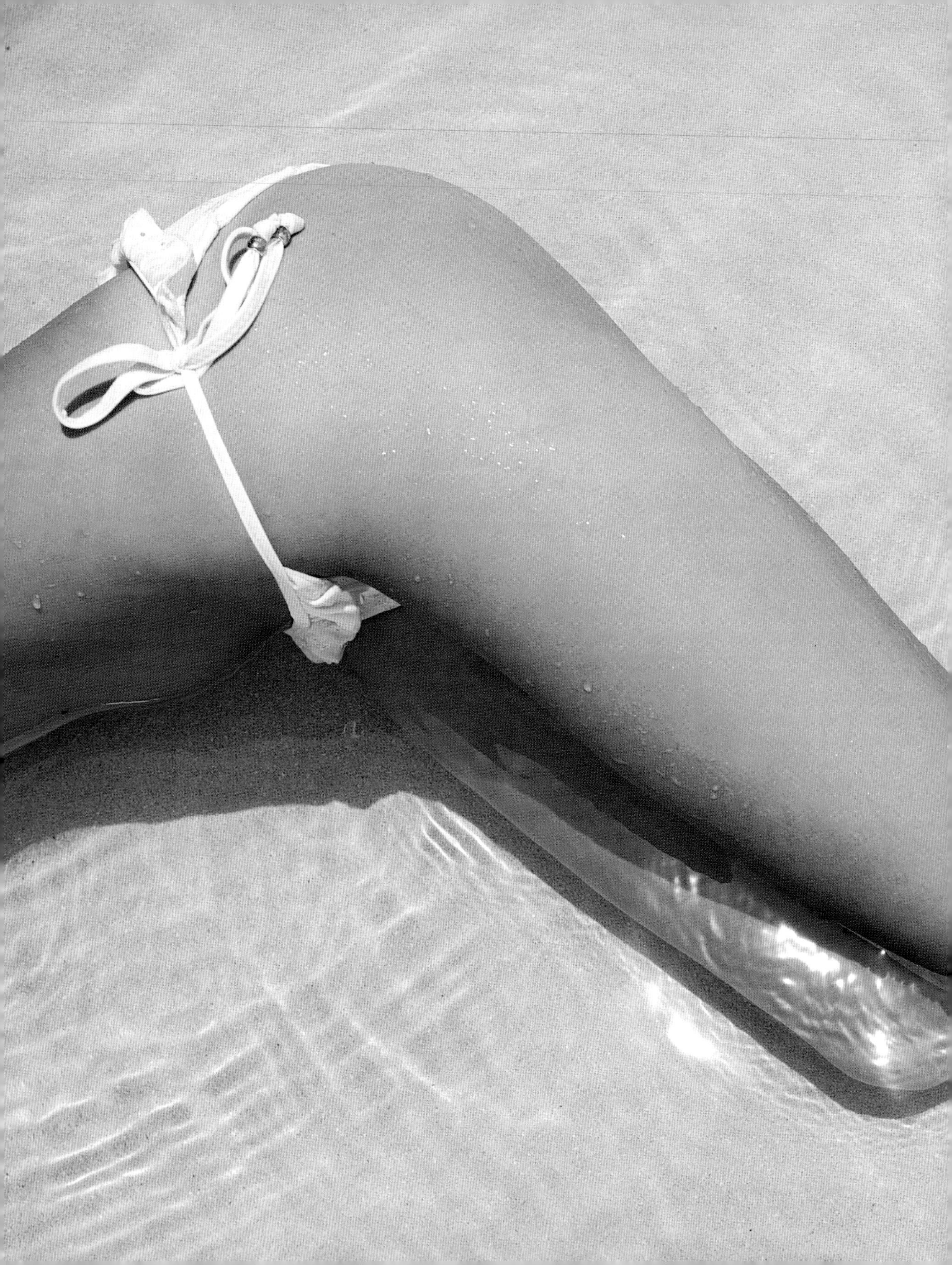

CHAPTER 3

CUT THE CRAP*

*THAT'S CAFFEINE, REFINED SUGAR, ALCOHOL, AND PROCESSED FOODS

THIS CHAPTER WILL REVEAL...

WHY TOO MUCH COFFEE WILL MAKE YOU FAT

WHY ALCOHOL SHOULD BE AVOIDED

WHY PROCESSED FOODS ARE SO HARMFUL

WHY YOU SHOULD AVOID BREAKFAST CEREALS

The four main toxins that cause our bodies to cling to fat are: Caffeine, Refined sugar, Alcohol and Processed food. Or CRAP. There are plenty of other causes, which we'll discuss throughout the book, but these four are the big baddies, and when a client walks through my door, these are the ones I warn them about straight away. For a quick, so-easy-you-don't-even-need-to-think-about-it guide to staying slim, just think: I must avoid CRAP.

C IS FOR CAFFEINE

Although caffeine is the first toxin I deal with here, it's actually the least fattening and most beneficial of the big four. This is because it is not so much caffeine itself that is so bad for you—it's the way that most of us drink it that's the problem. Excess caffeine (more than two cups of tea or coffee a day) stimulates your nervous system, causing your adrenals to pump out cortisol, a hormone which helps the body respond to stress. All that extra cortisol floats around your system for hours after you've drunk caffeine. So people who are drinking coffee or tea all day long are basically flooding their bodies with fat-storing stress hormones.

Then there are the calories that come from what I call "junk caffeine." That's coffee or tea with added sugar, or the iced coffees that come with flavored syrups or whipped cream. Caffeine past lunchtime can also disrupt the way you sleep, and a lack of good-quality sleep encourages your body to store fat, especially around your middle. But you should avoid decaffeinated coffee too because the caffeine-removal process strips it of a lot of its goodness.

Having said all that, I love coffee just as much as the next person. But I use it to my advantage: caffeine can help the body burn fat and it also boosts your performance when you're exercizing (have it at least half an hour beforehand). Organic coffee is also packed with antioxidants, and it's great for your digestion, helping to get your bowels going in the morning, keeping your body nice and clean and toxin-free. So go for one or two cups of organic coffee (or tea) a day, preferably in the morning. I love an espresso with a splash of full-fat organic milk or even cream; I also like a sprinkle of cinnamon on the top—it helps your body burn fat more efficiently and keeps blood-sugar levels steady. And the hit of flavor takes away the need for sugar and sweeteners.

Green tea also contains caffeine but less than coffee, so you can have more of it (up to six cups a day) and it also has more antioxidants. Plus it's a great detoxifier for the body. It's especially good at getting rid of metal toxicity—that's basically toxins from the environment. Start drinking it first thing and stop at around 5 or 6 p.m. I tell my clients to brew a big pot of it, wait for it to cool down, then transfer it into a bottle and drink it cold throughout the day.

Opposite is my "Bad, Better, and Best" guide to caffeine; always choose from the Best column if you can, or the Better column if you must. And unless you want a fat mid-section, avoid the Bad column altogether.

R IS FOR REFINED SUGAR

I've already explained why sugar makes you fat and tired (see pp. 25–26), ditch it if you want to become strong and lean.

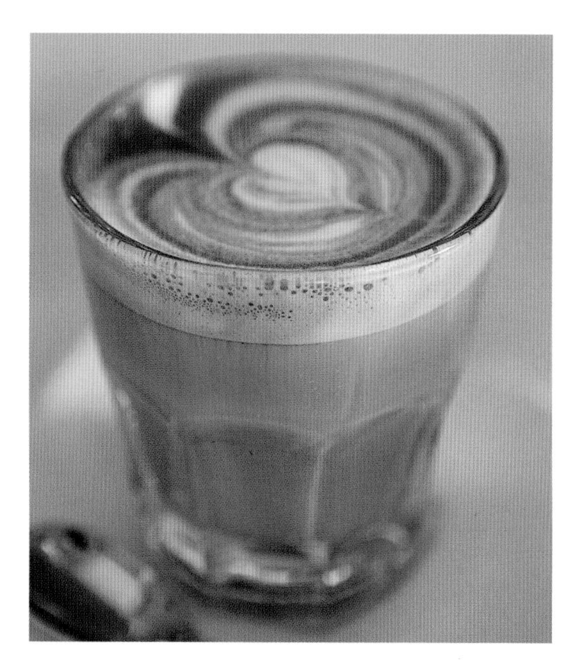

BAD	BETTER	BEST
Instant coffee—highly processed and full of toxins that clog up your liver and rob your body of nutrients	**Espresso**—a good quality organic coffee is full of antioxidants and can raise your energy, great about half an hour before an exercise session	**Espresso with organic cream**—a small, intense amount of good-quality coffee, and the cream will help keep you full and avoid sugar cravings
Black tea—fine in theory, and full of antioxidants, but there are healthier options	**Green tea**—great for speeding up your metabolism and full of health-boosting antioxidants. Plus the caffeine helps keep you alert	**Caffeine-free herbal tea**—peppermint, ginger, etc—a great detox drink and great for banishing cellulite
Milk chocolate—high in sugar and has very little antioxidant content	**Dark chocolate**—more cocoa satisfies your chocolate craving sooner	**Organic dark chocolate with nuts**—added protein slows the digestion of the sugar, preventing an energy crash
Fizzy cola (any brand)—full of sugar, preservatives and E numbers	**Sparkling fruit juice**—free from artificial sugar	**Sparkling water with a squeeze fresh lime**—super-alkalizing and contains no artificial sugars
High energy drinks—full of processed sugar and actually raise your stress levels—pretty nasty stuff in my opinion	**Guarana drink**—guarana fruit contains about twice the caffeine found in a coffee bean so is a more natural source of caffeine compared to high-energy drinks that are packed with chemicals	**Espresso with organic cream**—the cream makes the caffeine last for longer to make it a better fat burner
Shop or café-bought iced coffee—usually packed with sugary syrups and full of fat	**Espresso blended with ice and milk**—this way you know exactly what's gone into your drink	**Espresso blended with ground cinnamon, ice and organic cream**—cinnamon helps to regulate your blood sugar levels
Diet pills—nearly all contain some form of caffeine	**Green tea extract**—full of antioxidants, but as one capsule is the equivalent of about five cups of green tea, be careful of your caffeine intake	**Organic green tea**—super-high in antioxidants
Instant hot drinks (tea, coffee, hot chocolate)—processed and full of junk	**Espresso with double cream**—the cream slows the effects of the caffeine	**Caffeine-free/herbal tea**—full of antioxidants and helps fight cancer

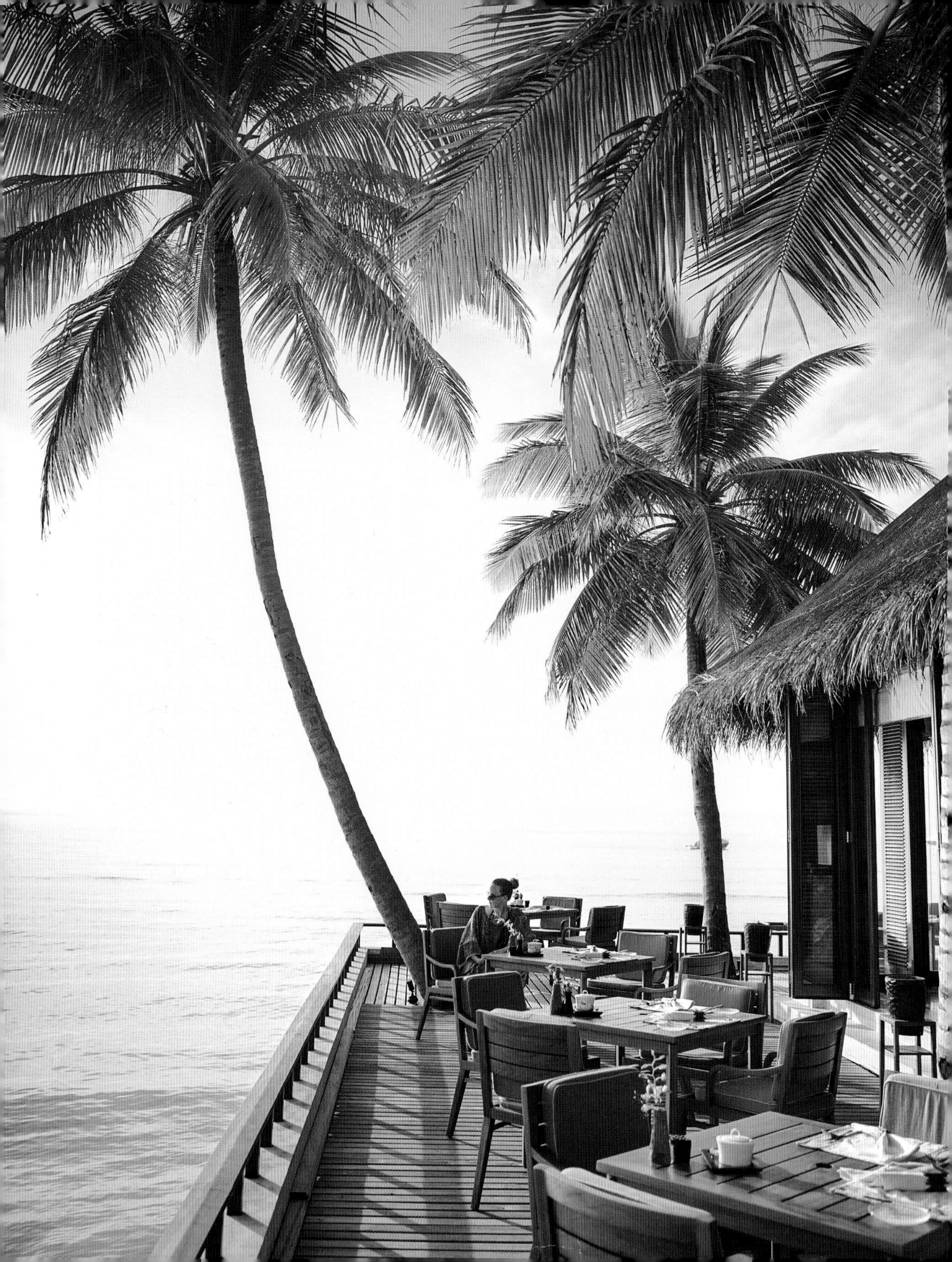

A IS FOR ALCOHOL

Alcohol is basically a poison and is just about as bad as sugar, and the only reason why I've spent more time talking about sugar is because we're exposed to it all day long, whereas most of us are only likely to drink alcohol in the evenings. For a start, it stimulates the production of foreign estrogen in your bloodstream, which promotes fat storage (again, around your waist and tummy) and decreases muscle growth. If you have lots of lovely lean muscle, your body will burn calories all day long and you'll look lean, toned, and amazing. But drinking alcohol will decrease muscle mass, leaving you squidgy and out of shape. It's no coincidence that studies have shown that women's waist sizes have got bigger over the years, in line with the amount of alcohol they consume.

Alcohol is the simplest and most fattening sugar of all. That's why it's such a good carrier of medicine—it hits the bloodstream straight away. During the 14-day Clean & Lean Kickstart, I want you to give up alcohol completely. And if you can't manage two weeks without alcohol, then this isn't the book for you, I'm afraid. You really do have to cut it out for two whole weeks, after which you need to change the way you drink (more about this in Chapter 10).

Nearly all my clients like a drink. I train businessmen who go out with clients every night of the week and play rugby at the weekends, so I'm used to dealing with people whose life includes alcohol. I know it's hard to cut back on beer and wine if your job involves wining and dining clients, but these are two of the least clean drinks you can have—clearer, lighter alcoholic drinks contain fewer toxins. But if you take in some of my changes, the results in your body will be amazing and it will be well worth it. So as a rule of thumb, I would recommend that you don't touch alcohol until you've reached your goal weight. Binge drinking on the weekend can take you two steps back, even after an otherwise healthy week; plus, a hangover makes you crave toxic foods... and smell nasty.

Remember also that your liver is a fat-burning organ. So when it's busy trying to process a large glass of wine, it can't metabolize all the calories you've consumed during the day. That means for every drink you have, you're slowing down your metabolism, so your body isn't burning any fat. In fact, it's the reverse: it's storing it. Alcohol is like a fat bomb that explodes all over your body, especially over your stomach, waist, thighs, and backside.

Some of my clients say, "But surely red wine has some health benefits?" Well, the answer is yes and no—but mainly no. Red wine does contain a very small concentration of antioxidants (from the red grape skins; so pick red over white), but there are so few of these in a glass that it's hardly worth it. You'd have to drink so many bottles of red wine to get any benefits that the alcohol content would far outweigh the goodness anyway. If it's antioxidants you're after, you're far better off just grabbing a handful of red grapes (or any other food that's rich in antioxidants for that matter).

BEER DRINKING MEN ARE TURNING INTO WOMEN!

Beer is one of the most womanly, girly drinks there is, and when men drink too much of it their bodies become flooded with the female hormone estrogen. This results in fairly slim, undefined arms, a huge round belly and "moobs" (man boobs). Many of my male clients arrive at my gym looking like this, and nothing makes them give up the booze faster than when I tell them, "All that beer is turning you into a woman!"

THE BENEFITS OF AVOIDING ALCOHOL

* You'll become slimmer!
* You'll look younger!
* You'll have more energy!
* Your stomach will become flatter!
* You'll become smarter!
* Your fertility will be improved!

So alcohol, we've established, has few health benefits. However—and as a non-drinker it's hard for me to say this!—I realize that most of you will want an occasional drink once you've completed the 14-day Kickstart. So overleaf is my "Bad, Better, and Best" guide to keeping it slightly healthier:

BAD	BETTER	BEST
Beer—the number-one fat-causing alcoholic beverage in the world—packed with sugar, yeast, and alcohol!	**Organic beer**—fewer pesticides and additives, meaning less stress on your liver (so a cleaner system); it's still loaded with calories though	**Vodka, mineral water, and a squeeze of lemon or lime**—the juice adds some nutritional value
Wine—packed with sugar, yeast, and alcohol	**Organic wine**—see above	**Gin and tonic with fresh lime**—a clean, yeast-free spirit with minimal calories
Alcopop—packed with sugar and alcohol, these are designed to taste like soft drinks, so you drink yourself fat without noticing	**Vodka and juice** (from concentrate) —a lot less sugar than an alcopop	**Vodka and freshly squeezed juice**—alcohol with some nutritional value
White wine—packed with sugar, yeast and alcohol	**White wine spritzer**—less sugar and less alcohol	**Vodka and mineral water with fresh lemon or lime** (see above)
Beer (see above)	**White wine**—less sugar than beer	**Red wine**—has some antioxidant properties
Cocktails with cola mixers, such as Long Island Iced Tea—packed with sugar, fattening amounts of alcohol, plus caffeine	**Cocktails with fruit mixers**—fewer bad sugars and calories, so less of a fat bomb	**Mocktails**—non-alcoholic cocktails made with freshly squeezed juice—full of vitamins, though still high in fructose/sugar
Vodka cocktails mixed with high energy drinks—equivalent to four coffees, plus a shot of alcohol; places your internal organs under stress	**Vodka and lemonade**—still too sugary, but at least you avoid the excess caffeine	**Vodka and mineral water** with a squeeze of lemon or lime (see above)
Shots with a milky liqueur and dark spirit e.g. B52; packed with sugar, alcohol, and dairy—a sugary fat bomb	**Single shot of clear spirit**—one poison instead of several; also, less sugar	**Shots are the beginning of the end!**—you really don't need them and your body will thank you for it in the morning if you just give them a miss
Malibu and cola—sugar with more sugar, plus caffeine and alcohol, and then some more sugar	**Malibu and pineapple juice**—some natural sugars, but still a fat bomb	**Vodka with freshly sliced pineapple**—a clean spirit with plenty of nutrients and a little bit of fiber; sip it slowly and enjoy the taste

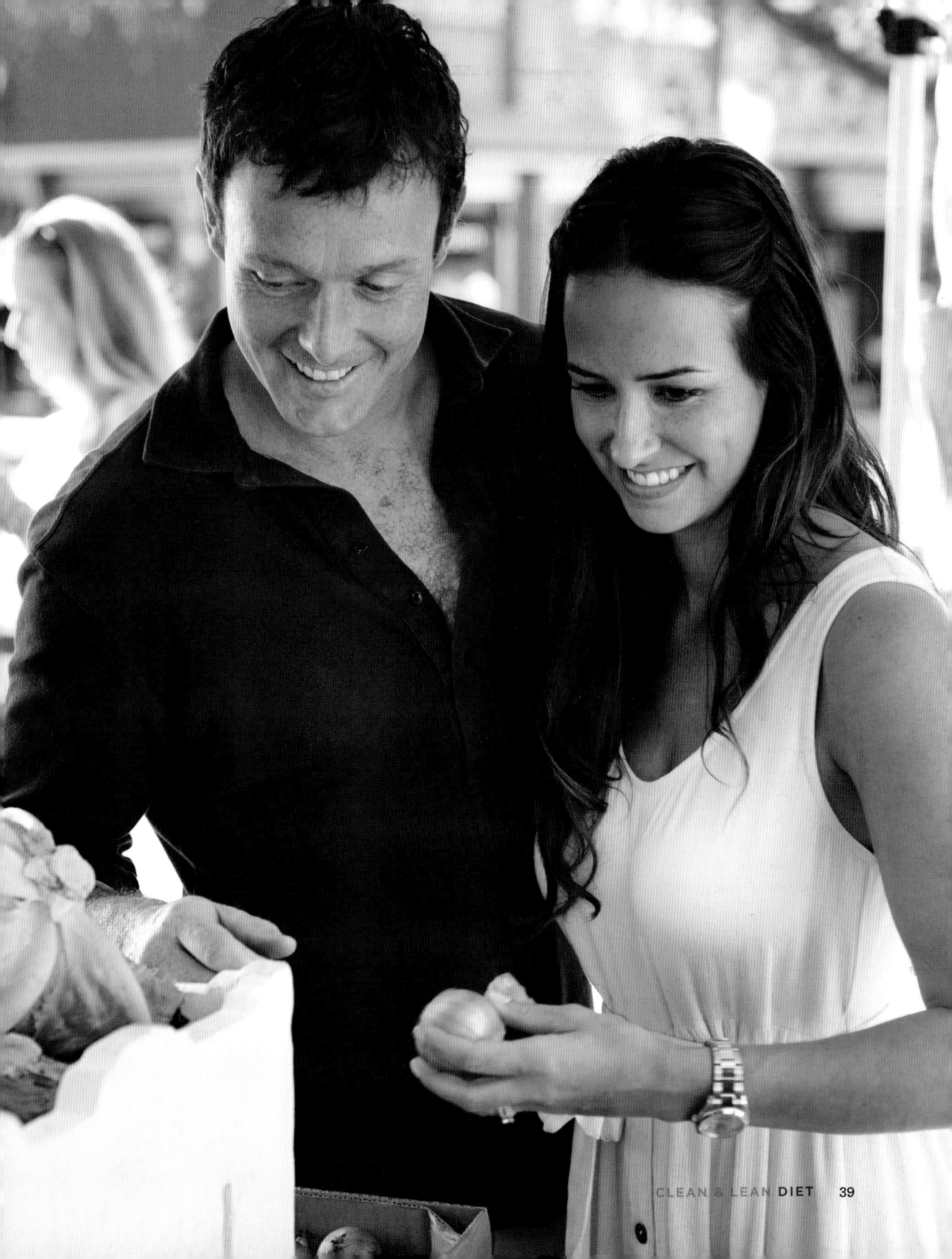

P IS FOR PROCESSED FOODS

A processed food is one that's been altered from its natural state to make it cheaper, more convenient, more attractive, or to extend its shelf life (or all four).

TRANS FATS

Always check food labels, as although trans fats are now less widely used, they can still be found in the following:

* Anything that includes the words "hydrogenated" or "partially hydrogenated" in the ingredients list
* Low-fat dairy products
* Margarines
* Doughnuts, cookies, muffins
* Processed meats
* Ice cream
* Salad dressings
* Ready meals

These go against every Clean & Lean rule there is. Clean foods are very close to—if not the same as—their natural state. Processed foods, on the other hand, are usually made in factories, stripped of their natural goodness, and pumped full of man-made additives and preservatives to make them look and taste appetizing and last longer. They became really popular in the 1970s when food manufacturers realized the financial appeal of mass-producing food that lasted a long time. It's much more cost effective for them to take average- or poor-quality food and process it, adding sweeteners, colorings and preservatives, than it is to produce fresh, clean food made from good-quality ingredients that go bad after a few days because nothing has been done or added to it to extend its shelf life.

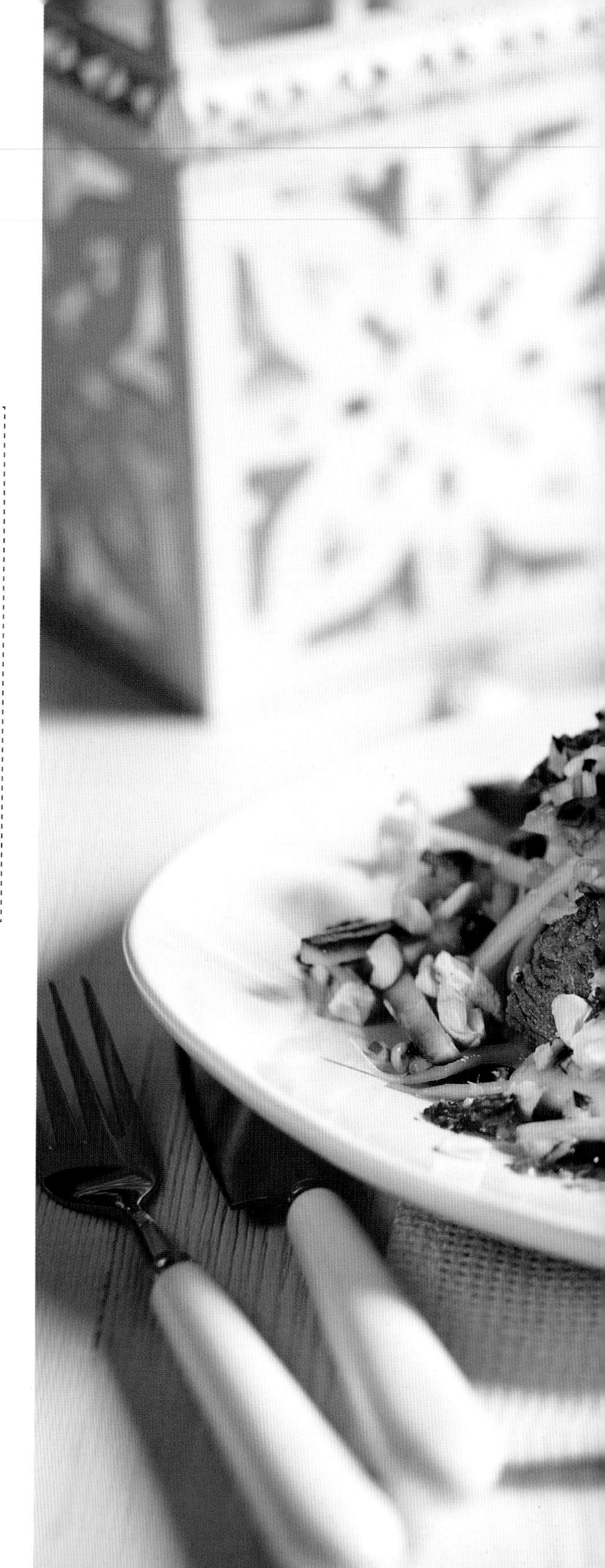

The following are the worst processed foods (in no particular order):
✳ Canned foods
✳ White bread and rice
✳ Processed meats
✳ Breakfast cereals
✳ Frozen ready meals
✳ Frozen french fries, wedges, etc.
✳ Packages of dried pasta or fresh pasta
✳ Packaged cakes, cookies, muffins
✳ Chocolate, candy, and potato chips

An increasingly popular method of preserving processed food is to hyper heat it. But this means health-boosting vitamins, fiber, and minerals are lost. That's why fresh fruit is much healthier for us than canned fruit, which has been heated, losing much of its vitamin C along the way. Remember I said earlier that the more vitamins and minerals you get, the more nourished your body becomes? Well if you eat a lot of processed food, you won't be getting a lot of vitamins and minerals and, as a result, you'll feel tired and hungry. Scientists are also discovering more and more evidence to show that preservatives—found in nearly all processed foods—can even slow down our metabolism and interfere with our fat-burning hormones.

I dislike processed foods. I mean, I really, really dislike them. In my opinion they make you fat, sick, and hungry, and go against every Clean & Lean rule there is. I don't know about you, but I don't want to eat anything that's been stripped of its natural goodness and pumped full of man-made preservatives.

Unfortunately, however, just about everything from pasta, bread, and yogurt to processed meats (like ham) has been processed. Having said that though, not all processed foods are as bad as each other. White bread, for example, has been stripped of all its goodness and pumped full of salt, whereas a container of organic natural yogurt with just a few ingredients—while still processed—has retained a lot of its natural goodness. Equally, an organic pasta sauce made mostly of tomatoes is better than a sweet-and-sour flavored sauce containing about twenty ingredients, all with scary-sounding names. So when it comes to processed food, just remember: the less that's been done to it the better, and the fewer ingredients it has the better.

To help you negotiate the minefield, overleaf is my "Bad, Better, and Best" guide to processed foods.

BAD	BETTER	BEST
Pre-packaged cakes—these sit on the shelves for months with as much nutritional value as the box they come in; stay away from them	**A freshly made cake from a baker**—a step in the right direction, but still loaded with wheat, sugar, and yeast	**Wheat-free, sugar-free, dairy-free muffin from a health-food shop**—you'll get fiber and a natural sweetener in the form of fruit
Pre-packaged crêpes—white flour and white sugar packed with preservatives; a fat bomb waiting to explode	**Homemade pancakes**—better than shop-bought, but try to replace white flour with either rice or buckwheat flour	**Bodyism pancakes (see p. 87 for recipe) with berries and banana**—more easily digested and taste great
Regular chewing gum—too sugary, plus it tells your stomach to "prepare for food," thus giving you a false appetite. Want fresh breath? Why not just brush your teeth or eat parsley?	**Sugar- and aspartame-free gum**—a little better, but still sending false signals to your brain and stomach	**Chew on fresh mint or parsley**—herbs are nature's medicine and these will leave your mouth fresh and your body healthy
Packaged meal with no protein (e.g. an all-pasta dish)—packed with bad carbs, sugar, salt, and bad fats, as well as leaving you hungry soon after because of the lack of protein	**Packaged meal with protein (e.g. chicken or fish)**—a step in the right direction, but remember most meats in these meals are heavily processed and packed with preservatives	**A fresh, steamed packaged meal with meat, vegetables, and nuts or seeds**—not easy to find, but when you have no time or energy to make food, this is by far the best choice
Salami—the leftover parts of the animal (lips and butts), this is heavily processed and packed with salt, delivering very few nutrients	**Slice of beef**—at least you know which animal it is from!	**Organic, freshly sliced lamb with guacamole**—a complete snack of protein, carbohydrates, and healthy fats
Packaged salad—often dipped in chlorine to retain the color and sprayed with preservatives to give it a long shelf life—this food is nutritionally dead!	**Plastic wrapped vegetable, e.g. cucumber**—but avoid it where you can and opt for the unwrapped vegetable	**Raw, unpackaged organic vegetables from a farmer's market or similar**—this is as Clean & Lean as it gets
Salad dressing—packed with sugar, salt, and bad fats	**Balsamic vinegar and olive oil**—provides a great Clean & Lean flavor and good fats that help fill you up	**Cold-pressed extra virgin olive oil**—the least processed of all oils with the most nutrients and the most flavor; or use Udo's essential oil
Water crackers—thin, dead, baked pieces of white flour	**Spelt crackers**—wheat-free and usually topped with seeds, making a much better dipping biscuit	**Oatcakes with avocado and smoked salmon**—a complete meal with quality protein and healthy fat

BAD	BETTER	BEST
All sweet crackers—loaded with sugar, wheat, bad fats, and yeast with a pinch of salt; need I say more?	**Rye crispbread with cheese**—wheat-free alternative with a little protein and rich in fiber	**Oatcakes with avocado and organic chicken**—a complete wheat-free meal with quality protein and healthy fats
Pretzels—salted wheat; will leave you hungry and thirsty	**Organic oven-baked potato chips**—often less salt and fewer bad fats (still not great though!)	**Homemade sweet potato chips**—low-GI and loaded with nutrients and fiber
Canned soup—high in sodium and has less nutrient content	**Cardboard or plastic carton of soup**—preserves the freshness of the ingredients more	**Organic homemade soup with protein e.g. chicken soup**—no sodium and full of nutrients
Table salt—little mineral content and can cause water retention	**Celtic sea salt**—contains 82 health-boosting mineral elements	**Himalayan salt**—uncontaminated with toxins and pollutants
Ketchup—full of sugar and salt	**Full-fat mayonnaise**—contains omega-3's	**Organic English mustard**—naturally flavored with spices
Sweet chili sauce—contains sugar, salt and virtually no health benefits	**Hot sauce**—sugar-free and naturally flavored	**Organic freshly sliced chile**—rich in vitamin C

*top tip

A well-nourished body doesn't feel constantly hungry: if you thoroughly chew a Clean & Lean chicken salad full of all kinds of vegetables, you won't crave something sweet afterwards.

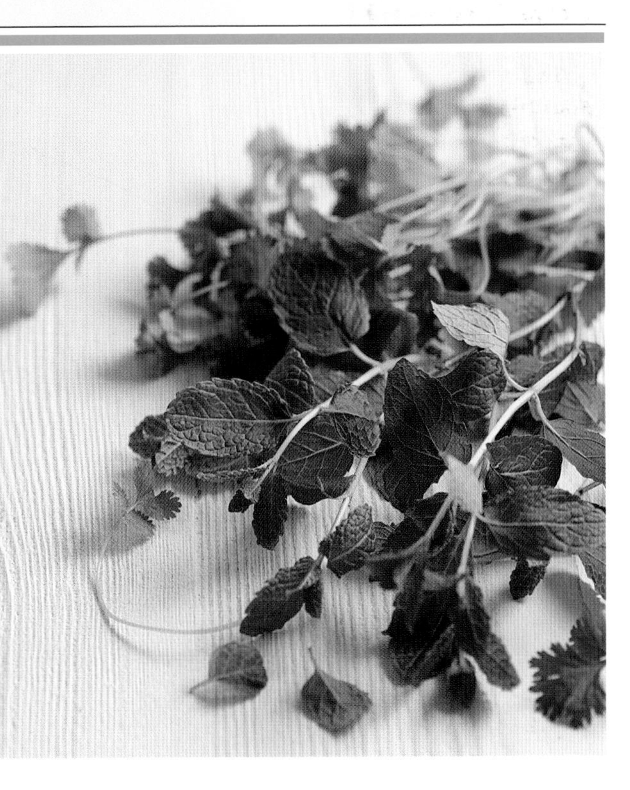

Don't be fooled by food labels

Processed foods sell well because of the clever marketing campaigns behind them. Phrases like "farm fresh," alongside pictures of lush green scenery, kid us into believing that a mass-produced food product made in a factory, using additives and preservatives, has come to us straight from the farm. We need to wise up, and not be fooled by the following:

Ethnic references

Tortilla wraps with Mexican flags on the package, for example, aren't necessarily made in Mexico. They are just there to make you think the food is exotic. It's more likely that they were made in a factory thousands of miles away from Mexico, using cheap white flour and other additives. And the same goes for curry sauces that make references to India.

Healthy claims

Be wary of products that claim to be low-fat, high-fiber, or reduced-sugar because there are no legal specifications for these claims. So if a product is labeled low-fat, it just means it has less fat than the standard version of the same product—it doesn't mean it's actually low in fat. The other problem is that if something is marketed as low-fat, it's often high in sugar, which is even worse. Processed cereals are a good example—yes, they're marketed as "low-fat" or "high-fiber," but food manufacturers add extra sugar to make them more palatable.

"Fruit flavor" drinks

There is probably no fruit in these. A drink or yogurt may be labeled as "strawberry flavor" without having to contain any strawberries. However—and this is where it gets confusing—if it's described as "strawberry flavored" (i.e. with an "ed" on the end), then most of the flavor has to come from real strawberries. It will still be heavily processed though, so stick to drinks described as "pure fruit juice" or just squeeze your own juices at home with a juicer.

Emotive descriptions

What do words like "ocean fresh," "country style," and "farm style" really mean? Absolutely nothing, so ignore them.

Healthy ingredients

A product says it contains goji berries or pomegranate, does it? Well, check the ingredients list—you may find it only contains a tiny amount of these ingredients, with a lot of processed sugar coming higher up the ingredients list.

What about processed carbs?

I'm not a fan of low-carb or no-carb diets as they tend to be restrictive, unsustainable, and just plain miserable. However, I do ask my clients to avoid processed carbs, which means most breads, pasta, and rice. Carbs are fine—I eat them all the time—but only in their most natural state, which means vegetables and fruit. There are some processed carbs which are OK—oatcakes, for example, or certain clean, lean breads, like rye. There are so many healthier alternatives to regular bread out there. So instead of white, brown, or multigrain bread (all of which contain lots of wheat; see below for why this is bad), try rice cakes, rye bread, sourdough bread, corn bread, or rice bread instead. Look for them in the health-food section at the supermarket or, better still, at your local health-food shop. And remember always to have protein with your carbs—even good carbs are still fairly high in sugar, so it's important to have some protein with them to slow the rate at which the sugar hits your bloodstream.

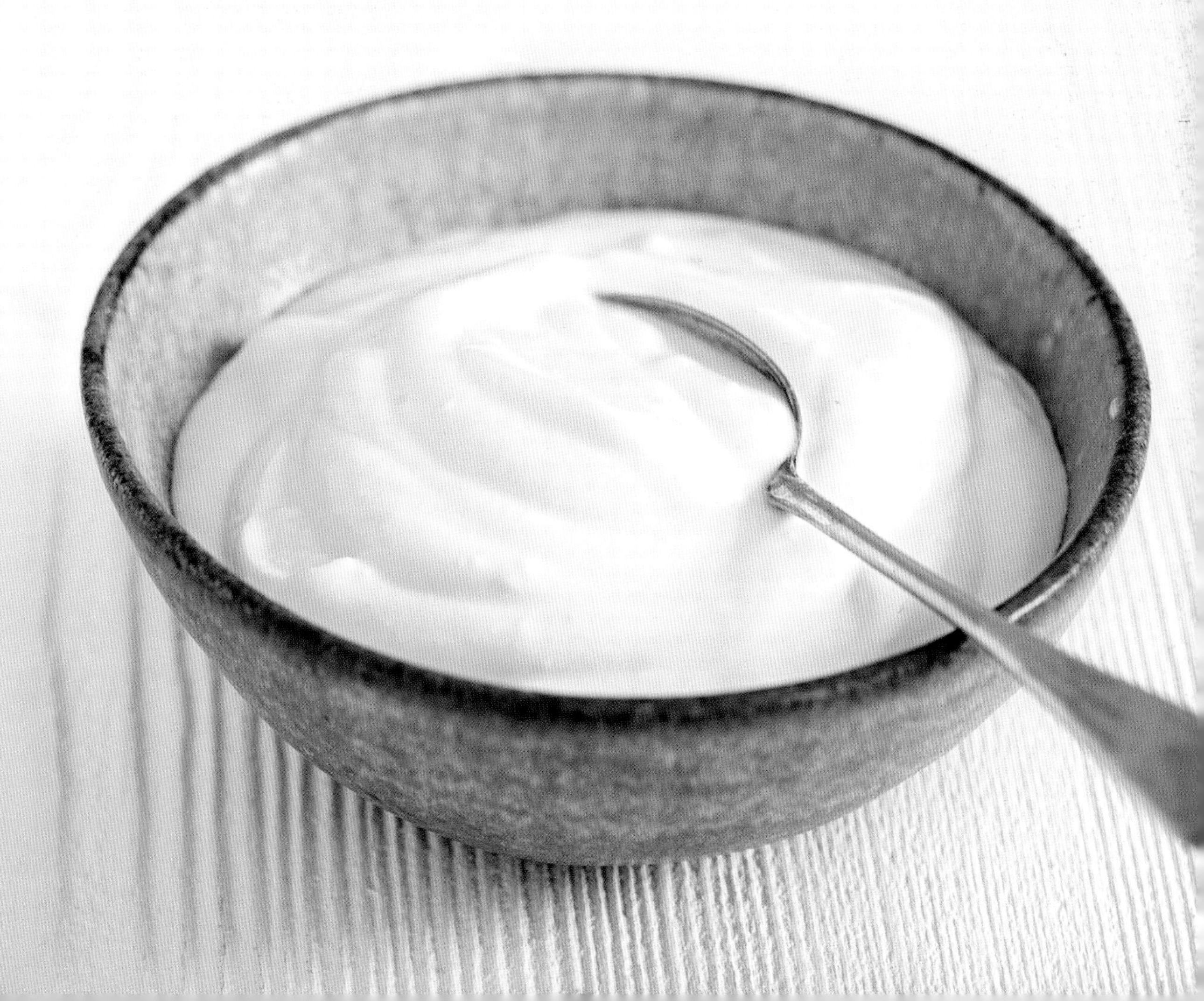

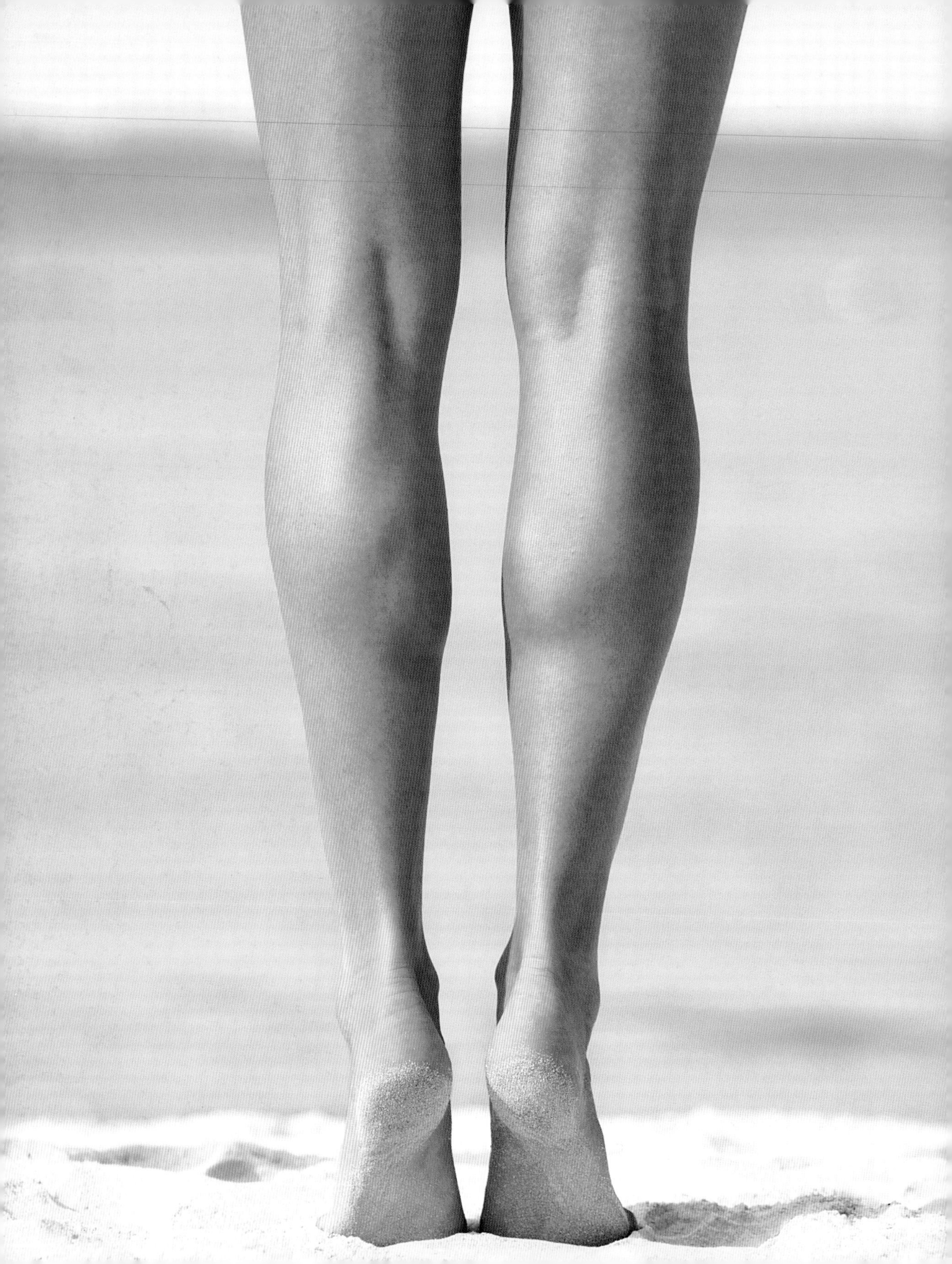

WHERE'S THE WHEAT?

By cutting out wheat and gluten, and all foods containing them, you'll lose weight and your stomach will become beautifully flat. However, it's hard to avoid them completely, so do your best by avoiding the following:

* All commercial breads
* All commercial breakfast cereals
* Pasta
* Muffins
* Pastries
* Baked goods
* Pizza bases
* Pie crusts
* Crackers
* Cakes
* Croissants
* Bagels
* Alcohol made from grains—i.e. beer, whiskey, and liqueurs
* Canned meat containing preservatives
* Canned vegetables (unless canned in water)
* Cheese spreads
* Chewing gum
* Commercially prepared soups
* Couscous
* Curry powder and seasoning mixes
* Desserts containing grain (stabilizers made from gluten)
* Horseradish creams/sauces
* Ketchup
* Processed meats
* Margarine
* Monosodium glutamate (MSG—found in many fast foods)
* Mustards (traditionally made with wheat flour)
* Salad dressings
* Sausages
* Semolina
* Soy sauce and most Chinese sauces
* White pepper in restaurants

And can I eat pasta?

Pasta is incredibly high in wheat (see below), so it can make you fat, sluggish, and bloated. Don't be fooled by whole wheat pastas either—they contain just as much wheat.

If you really love your pasta, look for the following alternatives: vegetable pasta, rice pasta, corn pasta, millet pasta, spelt pasta, buckwheat noodles, or quinoa. My beautiful wife Chrissy's favorite is brown rice pasta with pesto.

Remember!

Food manufacturers will try to trick you by using less obvious names for wheat, such as corn starch, edible starch, food starch, modified starch, rusk, thickener, or vegetable protein.

Avoid wheat—especially breakfast cereals*

Throughout this chapter I've mentioned "wheat-free" this and "wheat-free" that. But what's so bad about wheat?

Well, wheat and wheat products (found in so many processed foods) convert to sugar faster than any other grain. And don't forget, sugar converts to fat, so the wheat you eat will very quickly end up as fat all over your hips, thighs, bottom, and stomach. Most breads, pasta, and breakfast cereal consist mainly of wheat, which is why you need to limit them if you want to get a lean and lovely looking body.

Wheat also contains phytates. Phytates bind with health-boosting calcium, iron, magnesium, phosphorus, and zinc in the intestinal tract, preventing these minerals from being properly absorbed. If you eat wheat excessively, you could end up with mineral deficiencies (which make you hungry all the time), allergies (hay fever, skin rashes, and so on) and intestinal problems (such as IBS and bloating).

Nearly all products that contain wheat also contain gluten. Gluten is used mainly as a binder in the processing of food. Without added gluten, ketchup, for example, would be a runny tomato juice. Gluten can be very hard to digest though, and can in susceptible people cause indigestion, yeast overgrowth (candida), allergies, and celiac disease (a digestive disorder that affects the small intestine, causing bloating, diarrhea, constipation, and fatigue).

Do wheat and gluten agree with you?

If your stomach bloats out just below your belly button, especially after eating—what I call a "pooch tummy"—this is a classic sign of a wheat or gluten intolerance. Even very slim people get a little pooch tummy that sticks out if they're intolerant to wheat and gluten.

Why you need a wheat-free breakfast (most days)

For many of us, having wheat for breakfast is just a habit. There's no real reason to have toast or cereal first thing, yet so many of us do it out of sheer habit. I tell my clients to have something different though—like half an avocado sliced up on a few oatcakes or some oats, nuts, and seeds soaked in rice milk, try it, you'll love it! And more often than not, they'll look at me quizzically and say something along the lines of "Are you crazy?" Yet it's so much better for you to have a beautiful, creamy avocado on a crunchy oatcake than a bowl of sugary, salty, processed cereal.

And another great reason to ditch your regular toast or cereal: if you start having wheat-free breakfasts, you could be well on your way to having a lovely, flat stomach.

***Try these wheat-free breakfast foods:**

✳ Smoothies—use your favorite fruits, vegetables, rice milk, natural yogurt, chopped nuts, and seeds

✳ Eggs—poached, scrambled, or boiled, have them with wheat-free oatcakes or asparagus spears

✳ Protein—have a palm-sized portion of salmon (either smoked or a steak), chicken, fish, or even steak with something green (i.e, steamed broccoli, bell peppers, or zucchini).

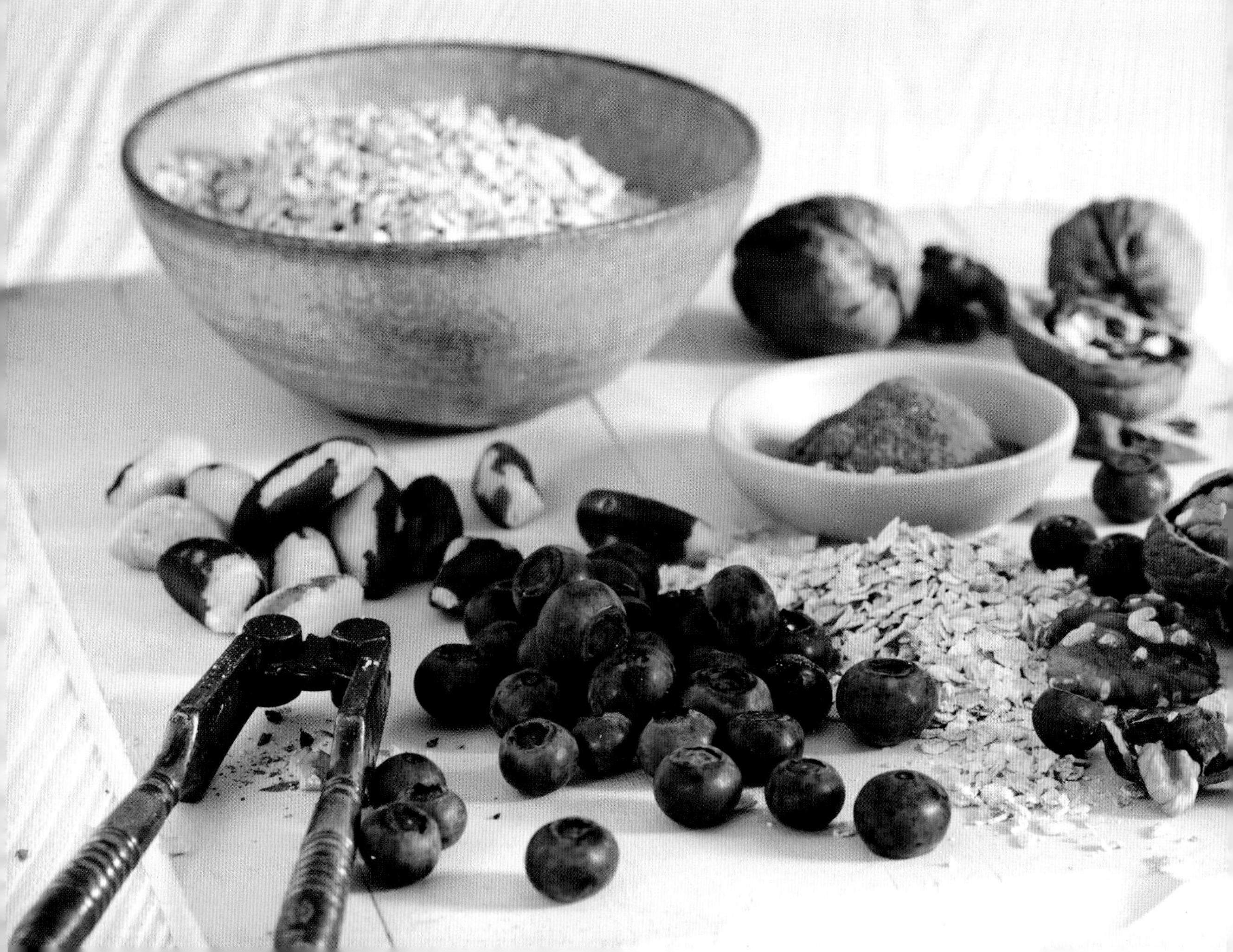

What's so wrong with breakfast cereals?

The majority of breakfast cereals (with a few exceptions) are far too high in sugar and salt, and are so heavily processed they could even be the C in CRAP. Check out the ingredients label of any breakfast cereal—sugar is often high up in the ingredients list, and this is the last thing you want at breakfast time. Why? Because it will cause a sharp increase in your blood-sugar levels. This, in turn, will increase the production of insulin, which will prevent you from burning fat and encourage your body to store it instead.

Something else worth noting is that cattle are fed on cereal because it's cheap and increases their body weight. Think about it: do you want to start your day with cattle feed?

Even cereals marketed as healthy options aren't what they seem. So ignore the ad of the girl in the swimsuit, or the sports star who tells you they never start the day without them (I don't believe for a moment an athlete would eat cereal unless they are a sumo wrestler—for one thing, their trainers wouldn't let them, if they're anything like me!) and just check out the ingredients. If wheat, salt, or sugar are on the list, put the box back on the shelf. Stick to lean breakfast foods like eggs, salmon, or avocado instead.

Overleaf you'll find my "Bad, Better, and Best" guide to carbs:

*top tip

Oatcakes are available at your local health food store.

*top tip

The darker and heavier the bread, the better. A good test when buying bread is to pick up a bleached, sugared, heavily processed white loaf in one hand and a natural, dark, dense loaf of bread in the other. The weight difference is enormous and the nutrient content is even more staggering.

BAD	BETTER	BEST
White flour—stripped of all nutrients, white flour also depletes the body of vitamin B	**Whole wheat flour**—slightly less processed and more fiber, however still contains gluten	**Any gluten-free flour**—coconut flour, rice flour, buckwheat, or millet contain no harmful allergens
Wheat-based cereal—most cereals are high in sugar and salt and heavily processed. Wheat converts to sugar very fast so will end up as fat	**Oat-based muesli mix with nuts**—more fiber than normal cereals	**Oatmeal with organic nuts and seeds**—low-GI, full of fiber and healthy fats
Wheat-based white pasta (most pastas)—pasta is very high in wheat and can leave you bloated and sluggish	**Whole wheat pasta**—contains fiber which will keep you feeling full for longer	**Rice and millet, corn, vegetable, or spelt pasta (gluten-free)**—a great alternative to wheat pasta
Cheese and ham croissant—full of fat and the energy won't last	**Wholegrain bagel with chicken and salad**—contains more fiber and also protein so will fill you up	**Clean & Lean lettuce wrap with organic turkey**—wheat-free and also free of toxins
Shop-bought low-fat muffin—high in sugar	**Oat-based muffin**—provides some dietary fiber	**Homemade muffin using gluten-free flour and raw honey**—no artificial sugars and gluten-free flour so leaves you feeling less bloated
Pre-made sandwich from shop made with white bread—processed, full of fat and probably packed with preservatives	**Rye bread sandwich**—rye bread is high in fiber and low in fat, and you can fill the sandwich with fresh Clean & Lean ingredients.	**One slice of rye bread with extra sandwich filling** (tuna, chicken, or meat)—reduce the amount of bread, and instead increase your protein
Tortilla—e.g. a burrito	**Hard-shell taco**	**Extra meat filling and salad (no taco)**—cut out the wheat altogether and up your protein
English muffin	**Wholegrain/multigrain bread** —high-fiber, but still too much wheat	**Rye bread**—more fiber and better for you
Jam doughnuts—full of sugar, wheat, and gluten; a recipe for storing fat	**Rye bread with organic strawberry jam**—wheat-free and contains fewer toxins, but still high in sugar	**Rye bread with organic nut butter**—full of healthy fats and dietary fiber
Pasta dish—pasta's high wheat levels will leave you bloated and sluggish	**Bolognese with rice**—rice is less processed than pasta	**Super Ground Beef (see p. 111) with quinoa**

BAD	BETTER	BEST
Couscous—too processed	**Brown rice**—gluten-free and rich in selenium	**Quinoa**—a superfood that provides protein and carbohydrates
White rice—a refined grain with little fiber	**Brown rice**—a good source of manganese and selenium	**Wild rice**—high in B vitamins and is a complete protein
Packaged waffles—full of sugar, salt, and all kinds of other junk	**Freshly made waffles**—much better than packaged, but still full of sugar and fat	**Clean & Lean pancakes (see p. 87)**—a great source of low-GI carbohydrate
Scones, jam, and cream—the processed sugar will leave you with a sugar crash and the scone may leave you bloated	**Scones and organic cream** (no jam)—cuts out the excess sugar, and the organic cream provides good fats	**Bran-based muffin with organic butter**—more fiber than a scone
Cookies—full of flour and sugar	**Rice cakes with nut butter**—high fiber rice cakes with the protein of nut butter	**Oat cakes with avocado and shrimp**—the perfect snack. The creamy avocado provides healthy fats and the shrimp provide protein
Potato chips—full of fat, packed with salt and artificial flavorings and preservatives	**Kettle chips**—still not healthy, but they have natural flavorings	**Sweet potato chips**—low-GI and high in beta carotene, a powerful antioxidant
Pizza bases—highly processed	**Whole wheat pizza base**—has a higher nutrient and fiber content	**Wheat-free pizza base, e.g. spelt**—free of allergens
Jam or cranberry condiment—packed with sugar	**Honey**—contains flavonoids which are a good source of antioxidants. Eat in moderation	**Organic nut butter, e.g. hazel, cashew, almond, pecan**—healthy fats and protein
Peanut butter (commercial), made with roasted, salted peanuts—processed, unhealthy, and full of artificial flavors and preservatives	**Unsalted peanut butter**—free from salt and hydrogenated fats	**Organic nut butter, e.g. almond, cashew, and macadamia**—full of healthy fats and antioxidants
Fries—deep fried, full of fat, usually coated in false flavorings and no nutritional value whatsoever	**Wedges**—one step closer to an actual potato	**Sweet potato wedges with shrimp and hummus**—natural and, with protein, a balanced meal

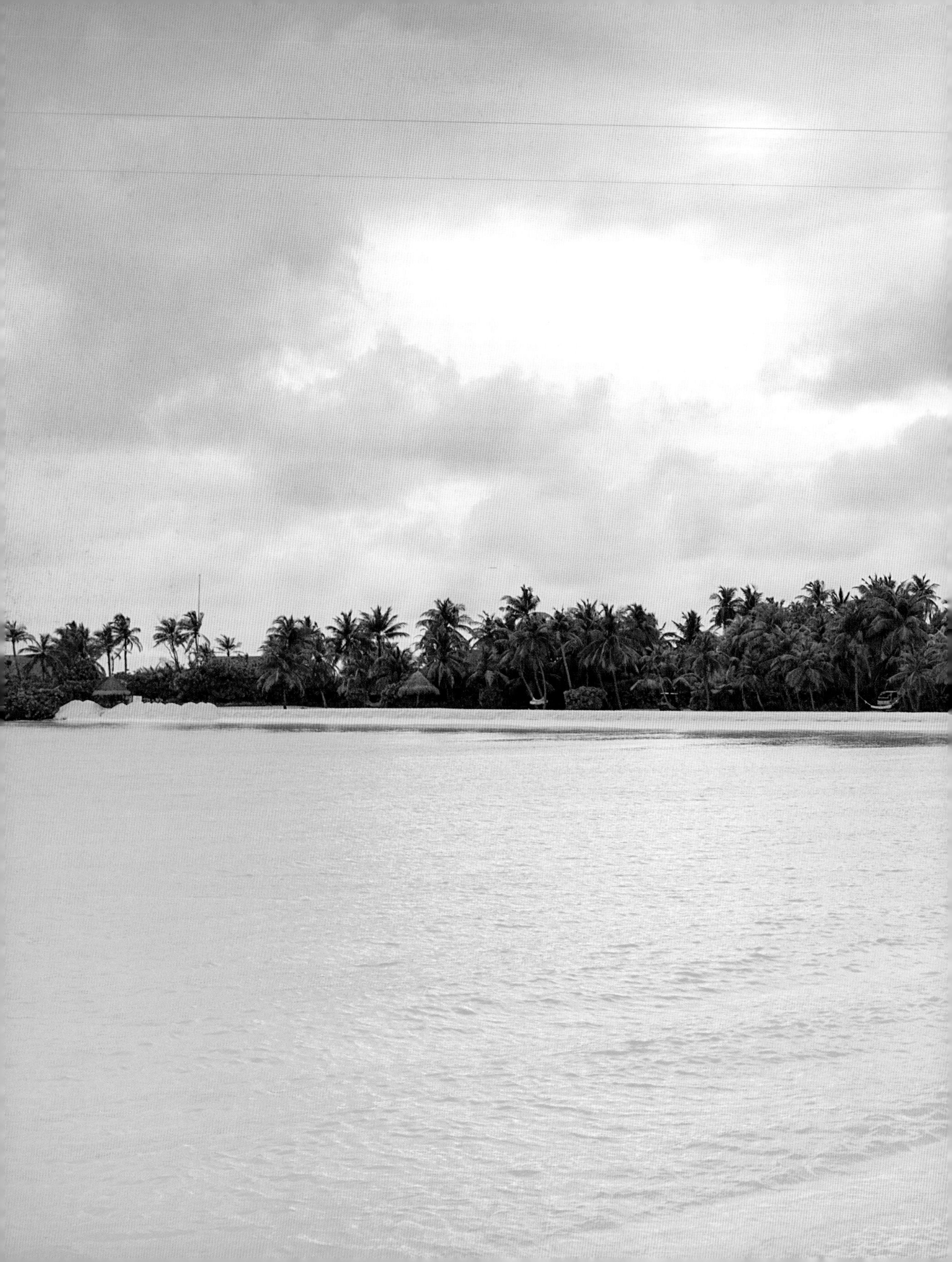

CHAPTER 4

WHY STRESS MAKES YOU FAT

THIS CHAPTER WILL REVEAL...

HOW DE-STRESSING CAN MAKE YOU SLIM

WHY TOO MUCH EXERCISE CAN MAKE YOU FAT

WHY HOW YOU EAT IS AS IMPORTANT AS WHAT YOU EAT

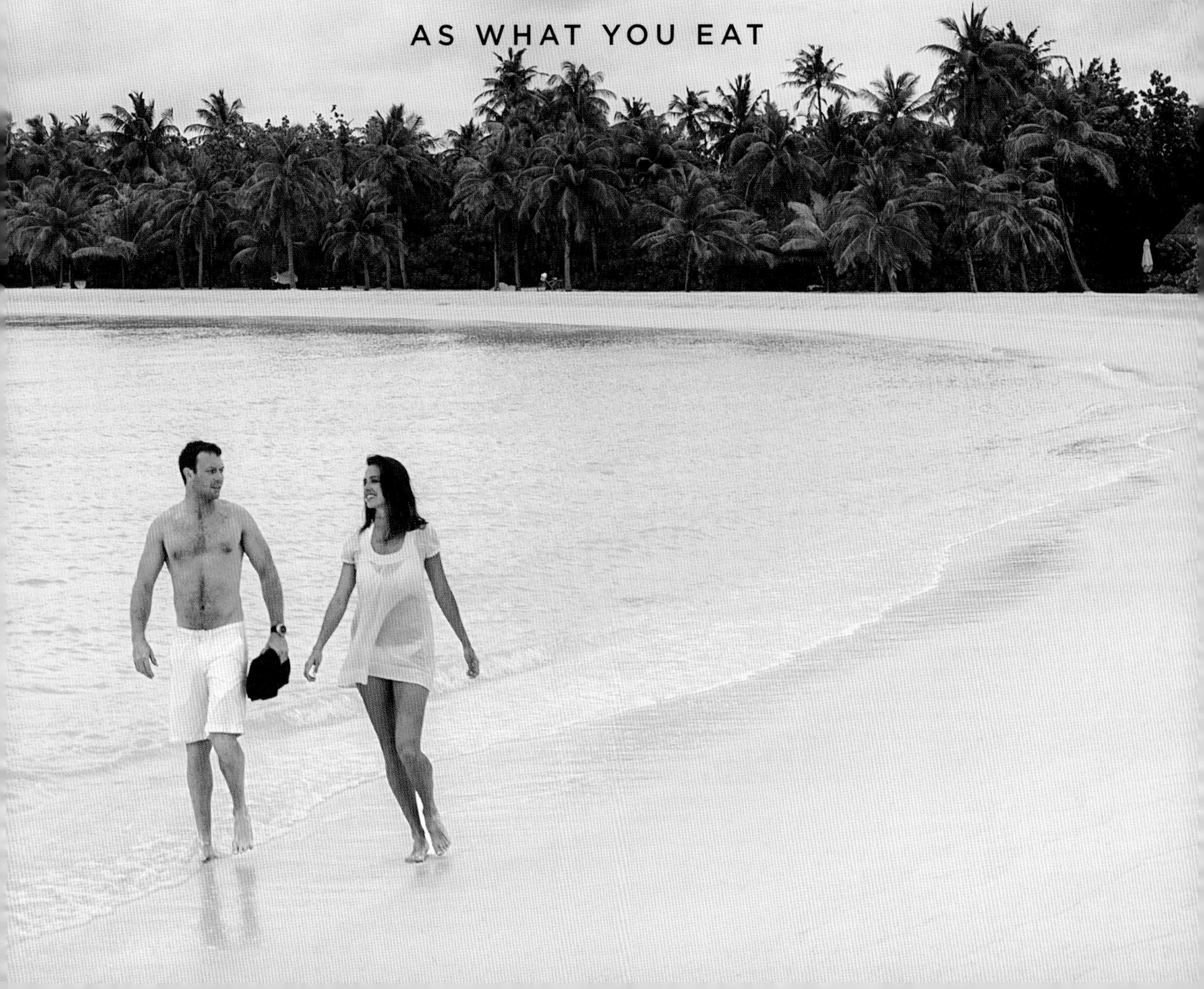

HOW DE-STRESSING CAN MAKE YOU SLIM

Aside from alcohol and bad food, stress is one of the biggest causes of excess fat. If you're doing everything else correctly (avoiding sugar, eating good fat etc.), but you're stressed, you will still have a fat little tummy and a thick waist.

When we're frightened, angry, tense, or worried our bodies become flooded with adrenaline and a stress hormone called cortisol (released from our adrenal glands—a tiny gland that sit just above our kidneys.) The adrenaline keeps us alert and focused, while the cortisol prepares our muscles for a "fight-or-flight" response. It's actually known as the "fight-or-flight" hormone because it gives us an immediate burst of energy which we can use either to "fight," i.e. confront a potentially harmful situation, or for "flight," i.e. to run away from it. It also helps the body to release sugar into the bloodstream for instant energy.

That sickly, jittery, panicky feeling you get in the pit of your stomach when you are stressed comes from the adrenaline and cortisol. It's all part of a defense mechanism that allows the body to respond appropriately when faced with danger and which was designed to keep us out of harm's way (especially in cavemen times when we had to run away from all kinds of dangerous animals).

Why modern stress is bad for you

While the stress mechanism worked well for us when we were cavemen, modern-day stress is not so good.

In fact, modern stress, caused by a relentlessly busy lifestyle, is really, really bad for you—even toxic. It causes you to get fat (I'll explain why below), it wears out your immune system and it increases your risk of serious illness. This is because many of the situations that cause you to become stressed nowadays aren't the sort of danger that you need to run away from—although your body still wants you to. While an important job interview, a looming deadline, or being told off by a scary boss may feel frightening, they won't cause you any physical harm, so there is no need for you to run away from them—which brings me to why stress makes you fat.

Why stress makes you fat

We've established that when you get stressed your body releases adrenaline and cortisol, and that when you're in real (i.e. physical) danger, these hormones prompt you either to run away or fight, in which case they don't make you fat. But when you're not in real danger, you don't use these fat-storing hormones, so they—and all that sugar that is released into the bloodstream—just float around, eventually ending up as fat around your waist. They also make you crave more sugar (in the form of chocolate and cookies) because your body thinks it needs more to keep it going. This is why stressed people often lose a couple of pounds on vacation—even though they may be eating the same amount as usual or sometimes even more, they don't have fat-storing hormones floating around their system every day, high blood-sugar levels or constant cravings.

The stress hormone cortisol is particularly bad for you. A 2011 study—published in the Journal of Obesity—found that women who reduced their stress levels lost the most belly fat. As stress levels subside, your adrenaline levels fall, but cortisol (and the resulting blood sugar) stays in the system much longer. Research from Yale University shows that fat cells around the stomach area have the most cortisol receptors, meaning they attract cortisol, giving you a layer of toxic fat just below your abdominal muscles that's really hard to shift. So doing regular sit-ups is going to be pointless if you always feel stressed—the only way to ditch this fat is to ditch the stress in your life. And remember—stomach fat is the most dangerous type of fat there is because it raises your risk of heart disease, high blood pressure, diabetes, and certain cancers.

Why stress makes you ill

As we've seen, the adrenal glands are the ones that release cortisol into the system. In many of my clients, these glands are overworked, making them unwell and overweight. Remember, they are meant for emergencies—like encounters with crazy animals or strangers in alleyways; they're not meant to be worked every single day. Yet many of my clients—probably like many of you—live in a world of constant, low-level, unrelenting stress: they oversleep; they rush around getting their kids (or themselves) ready for the day; they run out of the house with only coffee to keep them going (remember—coffee also causes your system to become stressed); then they face a day of late buses, traffic jams, deadlines, long lines, annoying colleagues, and so on. All day long, their bodies are being flooded with adrenaline and their poor, overworked adrenals are secreting cortisol to help them deal with all the stressful situations they find themselves in. They're literally running on empty and their systems begin to break down. Overworked adrenal glands can cause lowered immunity (resulting in constant colds and illnesses), tiredness, and fatigue. Sleep is affected too (if you've ever tried to fall asleep while the next day's to-do list is racing around in your mind, you'll know how true this is). Constant stress also shuts down the digestive system because your body redirects blood from there elsewhere (namely to your muscles). So stress can leave you constipated, bloated, and toxic. Beating this stress is the only way to better health and a better body.

Remember!

When under attack from stress, your adrenal glands also produce DHEA (dehydroepiandrosterone) which converts into estrogen, progesterone, and testosterone. That's why too much stress has a major effect on your sex hormones and can lead to a lower sex drive and fertility problems.

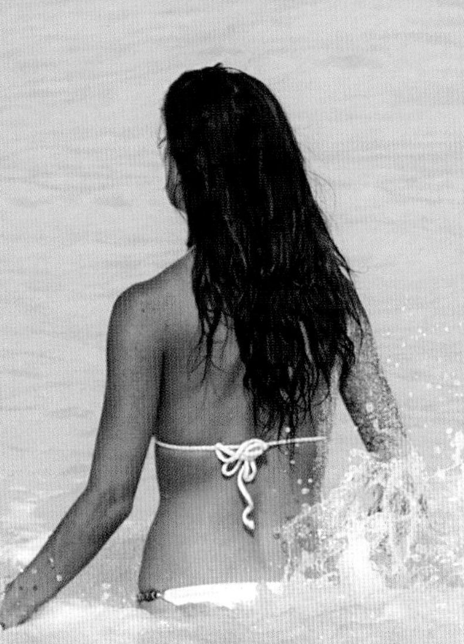

Why some foods make you more stressed

It's not just stress that makes you stressed—the wrong type of food does too. Potentially toxic foods—like refined sugar and processed foods (see Chapters 2 and 3)—will make you feel more stressed because they release sugar into the bloodstream too quickly. This increases the amount of stress in your body and also allows too much insulin into your system, which, in turn, plays a huge role in fat storage by making it harder for your body to burn off fat. Together, too much insulin and cortisol combine to give you a double whammy of fat storage plus increased appetite. It's a vicious cycle—the more stressed you get, the more you crave toxic food, which makes you more stressed, and so the cycle continues. Clean, lean foods, on the other hand, give you long-lasting energy, thus reducing stress levels. So break the cycle. Just chill out, don't exercise too much (see p. 57), avoid stress-inducing foods, and eat more stress-reducing ones (see p. 57).

LANNA'S STORY

"Over the last 4–5 years, my weight has fluctuated greatly. I put on weight easily and have always had an eye for the wrong sorts of food. I put on 26½ lbs when I moved from Perth to Sydney, mainly due to over-indulgence, and so I decided to start the big task of shedding all of those pounds.

It took me a long time to realize that a bad diet can't be out-exercised, and that my portion sizes were too big—I was never going to lose weight despite my valiant efforts at the gym! I tried various diets, and eventually found just enough success in time for my wedding. And yet slowly but surely, the pounds crept back on and ten months after my wedding day, I found myself 20 lbs heavier.

I was frustrated by the weight gain and by the way that certain foods would make me feel. I bought the *Clean & Lean Diet* book, as well as Body Brilliance and in such a short space of time, I lost 4½ lbs and inches from all over my body.

One of the main things I have noticed is the way I FEEL—my energy levels are higher and far more consistent over the course of the day and despite earlier mornings, harder workouts, and longer hours at work due to a promotion, I feel bulletproof, strong, and healthy!"

Stress-inducing foods

Candy—sugary snacks give you a quick burst of energy, but then cause your blood-sugar levels to crash, leaving you feeling sluggish, stressed, and with poor concentration. Avoid them like the plague.

Processed foods—these are full of junk and deplete the levels of vitamins and minerals in your body, leaving you more prone to stress. Stick to clean, lean, natural foods.

Junk food—studies show that foods high in bad fats (burgers, chips, etc.) lower your concentration levels and increase your stress levels. Hence that tired, jittery weird feeling you get after a bag of greasy junk food.

Salty foods—these increase your blood pressure, making you more prone to stress. The worst offenders are processed meats like ham and bacon, and processed foods which are full of salt.

Coffee—too much caffeine stresses out your system by constantly flooding your body with the fat-storing hormone cortisol. Stick to one or two cups of organic coffee a day.

Alcohol—this stimulates your poor, overworked adrenal glands. Go easy on alcohol to give them a chance to recover. Alcohol is also full of sugar which makes you toxic and fat. People mistakenly think it will help them to unwind after a hard day, but it has the opposite effect—it just stresses your whole system further.

MELISSA'S STORY

"The *Clean & Lean Diet* book completely changed my life! I am a mother of two who used to be the fussiest and most unhealthy eater. I was the type of girl who would binge on chips and chocolate and consume 2 liters of diet coke a day. I would constantly go on extreme diets, only to fail weeks later and continue on my old path. That is until I bought the *Clean & Lean Diet* book.

Something about clean eating really hit home with me. The way James wrote the book made me look beyond the short-term goal of weight loss and really think about not only my health but also the health of my family. All these years I was slowly killing my husband, my kids, and myself with an overdose of preservatives and sugar. I read the *Clean & Lean Diet* on a Friday and was so inspired I got up and threw away every boxed thing in my fridge and pantry and started my new way of life the very next day.

Now nearly ten months later I am happy to say that I have the healthiest diet of all my friends and family and I'm the go-to girl on nutrition and exercise. People comment on my weight loss and how radiant I look. Once I focused on nourishing my body with good food, the weight dropped off. But this was just an added bonus to my increased happiness and energy. I am so extremely happy and I thank James for helping me to change my life and my families' lives forever."

Stress-reducing foods

Berries—these are packed with vitamin C, which helps the body to deal with stress. Plus, they're full of fiber, which helps to regulate blood-sugar levels.

Green vegetables—dark green vegetables help to replenish the body with vitamins. Have these with every meal if you can, but make sure they're organic.

Turkey—this contains an amino acid called L-tryptophan, which releases serotonin (a calming, feelgood hormone) into the body. Eating turkey has a soothing effect on the body and can even help you sleep better. Keep it clean and lean by choosing skinless and organic turkey.

Sweet potatoes—they'll satisfy a carb craving, and contain more fiber and vitamins than white potatoes.

Avocados—they're creamy, so they satisfy cravings. Plus, all the good fat and potassium they contain can lower your blood pressure (and therefore stress levels).

Nuts—they help boost a battered immune system, plus they're full of B vitamins, which help to lower stress levels. Snack on a small handful, but don't go overboard with your portion sizes. Stick to a handful a day.

Bodyism Serenity—this stress-busting blend of vitamins, minerals, fiber, and protein is one of the best ways to kickstart your day. It contains magnesium to reduce cortisol levels and aid restful sleep (bodyism.com).

Why too much exercise can make you fat

I see lots of high-flying business people who are literally running themselves fat on the treadmill. Why? Because if exercising makes you stressed—either because you're doing too much of it or because you're running around to squeeze your gym classes in after work—then it might also be making you fat because of all the extra cortisol you're producing. People who go to the gym too often can still have slightly poochy stomachs, even when the rest of their body is well sculpted. If a new client tells me (proudly) that they go to the gym five or six times a week, I tell them to cut it down to twice or three times and to replace a cardio session (e.g. a run on the treadmill) with a yoga or Pilates session to calm them down and relax their system (see Chapter 9 for more on Clean & Lean exercise).

The benefits of eating properly

* Your stress levels will reduce.
* You'll look and feel less bloated.
* You'll feel fuller quicker, so you'll eat less at mealtimes and look leaner.
* You won't feel uncomfortably full or bloated.
* You won't mindlessly munch—when you stress-eat, you don't take time to listen to your body properly, so you often end up eating when you're not even hungry.

ZOE'S STORY

"I used to be the queen of quick eating but learning to chew has given me a flat stomach. I used to eat breakfast at my desk, which would usually be muesli that I would swallow half chewed. I'd often be so busy I'd eat lunch at 3 p.m., by which point I'd be ravenous. I'd grab a sandwich and eat it in less than 10 minutes before racing off to a meeting. I'd grab snacks all afternoon and eat them quickly too. Then, when I got home, I'd be in such a rush for food that I'd swallow down mouthfuls of pasta that I hadn't even chewed properly. I always felt bloated and my stomach stuck out like I was in the early stages of pregnancy.

James has taught me that no matter how busy you are, you can always put aside 20 minutes to eat something properly. I started chewing every mouthful thoroughly, which meant I could really taste my food. Within about two weeks, my stomach was completely flat."

Why how you eat is as important as what you eat

You can follow all the diet and exercise rules in this book to the letter, but if you're skipping meals, eating too quickly, or eating while stressed, you'll never be Clean & Lean.

One of the best things you can do for your body is to learn how to chew properly. Chewing is the cornerstone of healthy eating. So a salad, for example, is not really that healthy unless you chew it properly. This is because chewing releases all the vitamins and minerals contained in the food. It also produces saliva and breaks down food, so it can be more easily digested after you've swallowed it. If you eat too fast and swallow half-chewed lumps of food, they'll fester in your stomach and take longer to digest, resulting in bloating and wind.

What I want you to do is to take your time over every single meal. It should take you at least—at least—twenty minutes to finish a meal. More if it's a big meal. I want you to chew every single mouthful at least—at least—twenty times. More if you can manage it. I want you to chew each mouthful of food until it's a watery, mushy paste. And I promise this will have an amazing effect on your body.

How not to stress-eat

* Chew each mouthful at least twenty times—thirty if you can manage it.
* Put your cutlery down and take a few breaths between each mouthful.
* Don't swallow until your food is a watery paste.
* Only ever eat when you're relaxed. If you're stressed, wait until you feel better before eating.
* Stop when you're full and don't be afraid to leave food on your plate. You can always have more food later on, if you become hungry again.
* Don't mistake stress for hunger—if you're stressed you need to calm down, not eat.
* Make sure you're drinking plenty of still water—when you're stressed it's easy to forget to stay hydrated.
* Don't watch TV or do any type of work while you're eating. Focusing on something other than your food can lead to overeating.

YOU'VE PROBABLY GOT STRESS FAT IF

* you eat while stressed
* you are slim everywhere apart from your stomach
* you eat quickly
* you always crave sugary foods
* a bad day makes you hungry.

WHAT ARE YOU ACTUALLY HUNGRY FOR?

This is a question I tell clients to ask themselves when they're rooting through the cupboards for something to snack on. And, more often than not, they're not hungry for food; they're looking for a distraction because they're stressed, lonely, bored, or tired. All these emotions make you hungry for something—but food is not the answer. If you're stressed, you're hungry because your body is flooded with adrenaline and cortisol, which play havoc with your sugar levels, causing you to crave something sweet. But instead of reaching for the cookies, you need to take time out, breathe deeply, and work through your stress before you eat anything. The same goes if you're lonely or bored: find something else to distract yourself with—either a TV show, a movie, or a hot bath. Or you could be proactive with your body and do your 12-minute workout if you get hungry (see p. 134)! Eating won't cheer you up; it'll just provide a short distraction.

If you're tired, allow yourself to be tired. I'm constantly amazed at how many people don't let themselves wind down in the evening—they're always looking for a quick fix to prop up their flagging energy levels after work, whether it's a glass of wine, some chocolate, or a coffee. Allow your body to fall into tiredness and get an early night. Don't prop yourself up with a constant stream of stimulants.

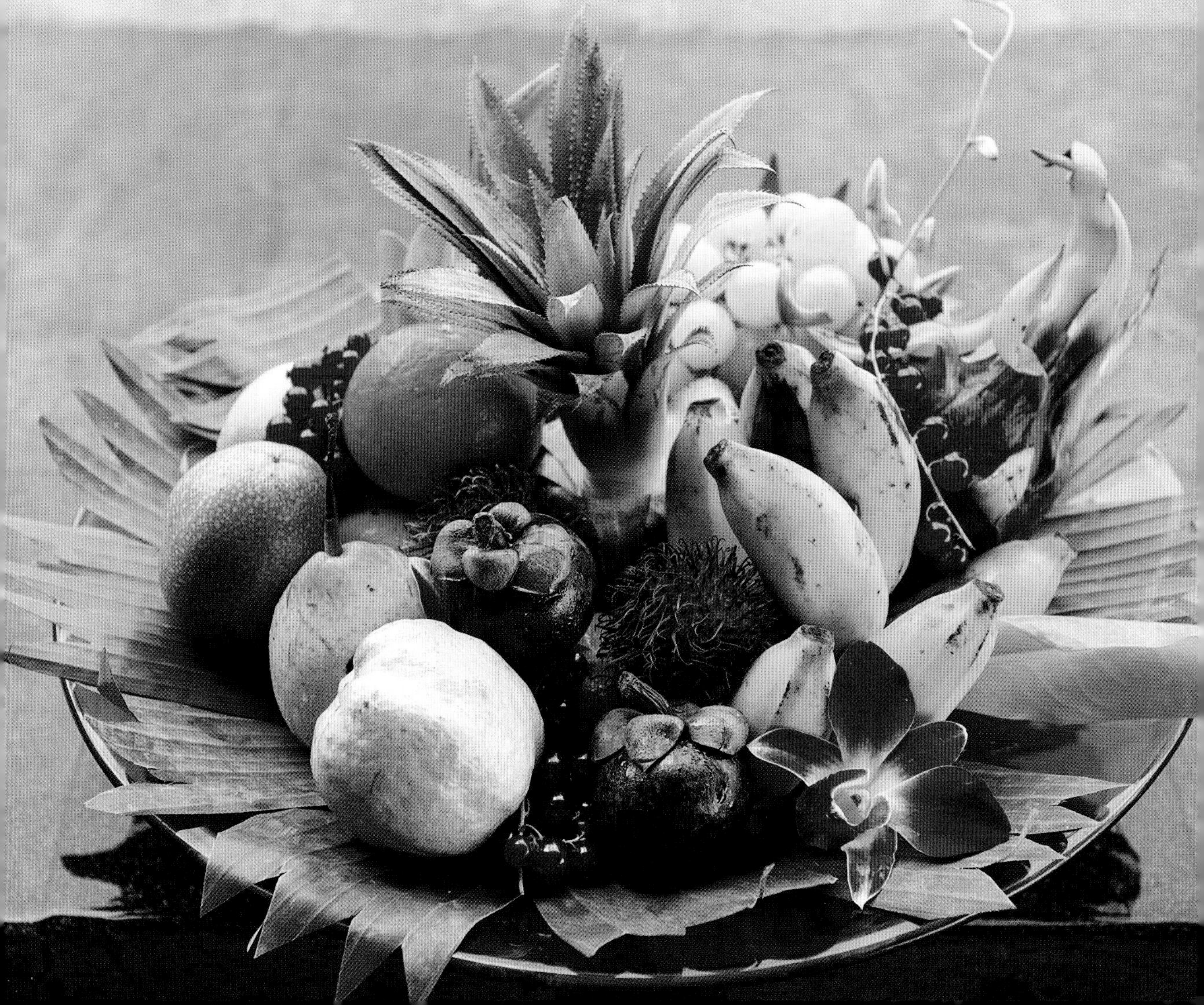

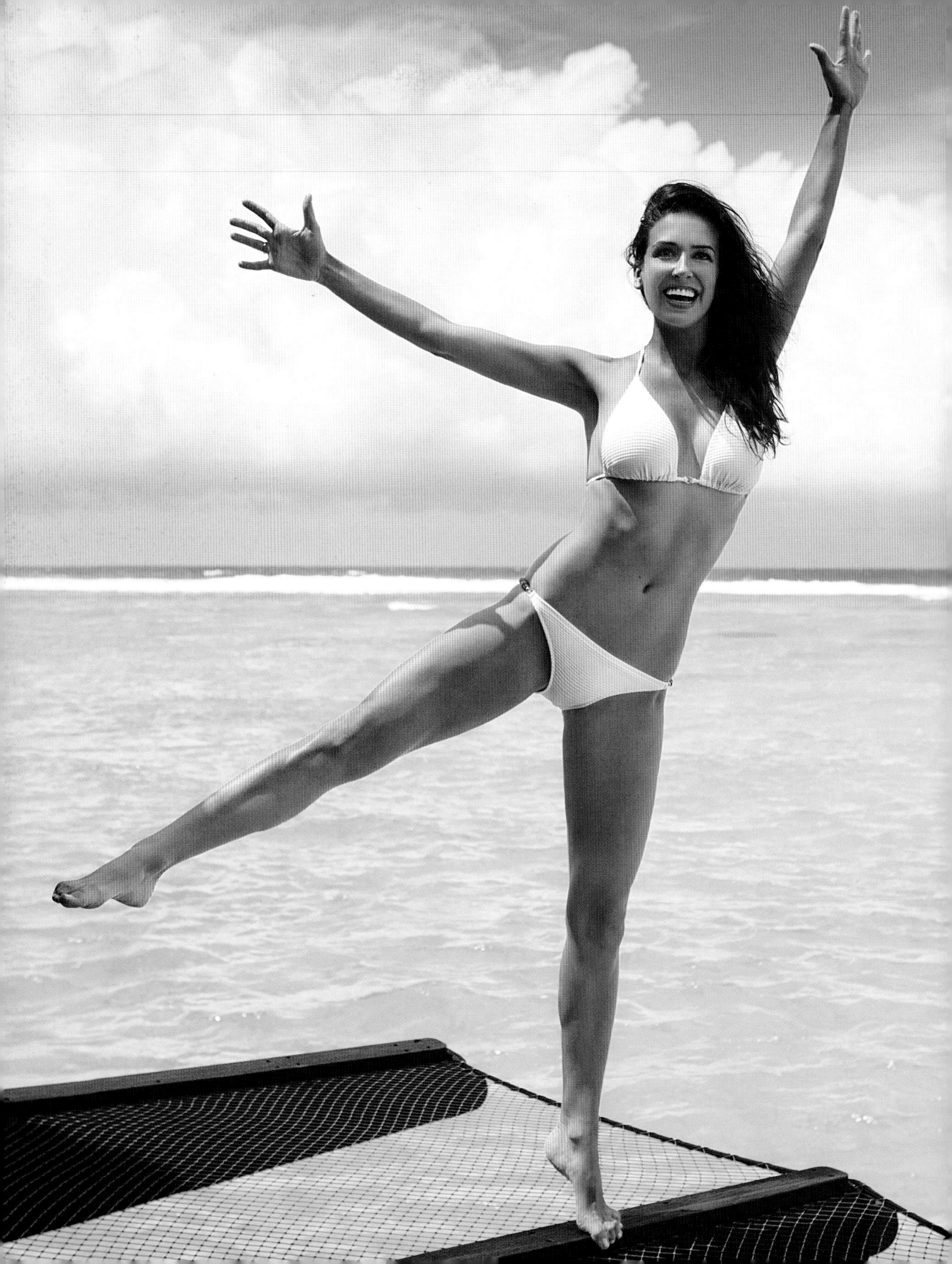

CHAPTER 5

WHY (GOOD) FAT MAKES YOU SLIM

THIS CHAPTER WILL REVEAL...

HOW FAT PHOBIA IS RUINING YOUR DIET

WHY (GOOD) FAT IS SO SLIMMING

HOW TO COOK FAT THE CLEAN & LEAN WAY

HOW FAT PHOBIA IS RUINING YOUR DIET

Growing up, it's drummed into all of us that fat makes us, well, fat, of course. Our moms went on fat-free or low-fat diets when they wanted to lose weight, and we took note. Fat was—and still is—seen as the big bad baddie. Its name alone gives it a bad reputation because it's associated with the fat sitting around our waist that we're desperately trying to shift.

ABBY'S STORY

"I have lots to thank Clean & Lean for. In 2009 I under went two operations for thyroid cancer. The second operation left me with damage to my parathyroids and as you can imagine this was not only scary, but it wreaked havoc with my weight and, after my operations and a lot of medication, I was heavier than ever.

However, the positive was that cancer had changed my priorities. I read a lot about lifestyle and health and started going to the gym religiously. It became the most important thing in my life and I was disappointed when I only lost 6½ lbs after a whole year of hard work. I thought I was doing everything right.

When I came across James' book, I lost 15½ lbs easily in 6 months. It was so simple. I am now at my goal weight and feel amazing. Now I recommend Clean & Lean to everyone. I tell them that with Clean & Lean, success is guaranteed."

But guess what? Fat doesn't make you fat. Sugar does, and so do bad carbs (both of which, ironically, are almost entirely fat-free). But fat? Absolutely not. In fact, eating good fat—as you'll learn in this chapter—will make you very slim indeed. It's like the anti-sugar. In the same way that sugar gives you premature wrinkles, makes you hungry, and causes you to gain weight, good fat will take years off your face, banish your hunger and cravings, and help you whittle down your waist. So don't be afraid of fat. But just to reiterate—I am talking about "good fat" here, not "bad fat." And I'll explain the difference later in this chapter.

When they first come to see me, nearly all my clients tell me proudly that they have very little fat in their diets. In fact, one of the biggest complaints I hear is: "I just don't get it, James. I have hardly any fat in my diet and buy low-fat or fat-free versions of everything, but I just can't lose weight." And I tell them it's because they don't eat any fat that they are fat. If they'd get over their fat phobia, they'd lose weight.

Why (good) fat is so good

First things first: not all fats are created equal. When I refer to fat, I'm talking about the good type—the type that makes you slim, young-looking, and energized. This type of fat is found in foods like nuts, seeds, oils, meat, fish, seafood, and avocados.

Good fat prevents you from overeating by telling your brain when to stop. You literally cannot binge on good fat because it fills you up so much. Don't believe me? Then try having half an avocado on some oatcakes for breakfast—you won't be hungry until lunchtime. Then, the next day, try having some low-fat cereal with skim milk

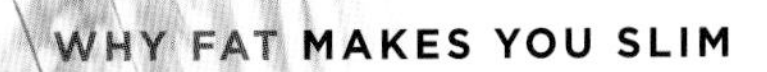

and fruit, or some toast and low-fat spread. Chances are you'll be hungry less than two hours later. This is why fat-phobic dieters are hungry all the time (and tired and miserable). There's something in good fat that switches on your brain's "stomach full" signals, and countless studies show that people who eat good fat every day are slimmer than those who don't.

For this reason, I tell all my clients that they must have some fat with every single meal and snack. It goes against a lot of what they thought before, but it works. So never eat anything without having a bit of fat with it: if you have some grapes, eat a few almonds at the same time; if you have a salad, add some avocado or organic goat cheese or even just a splash of olive oil. Never have a fat-free salad.

Fat slows the rate at which sugar hits your bloodstream, and this allows your blood-sugar levels to remain steady, keeping hunger and cravings at bay and leaving you slim and energized. So no meal or snack should ever be totally fat-free. I know I'm repeating myself here, but I can't stress enough how great you'll look and feel when you start introducing good fat with everything.

Good fat also burns fat and gives you a flat stomach and a small waist. Essential fatty acids—found in oily fish like salmon—help to shift fat out of the fat cells and into the bloodstream where it can be worked off by the body. Studies also show that these fatty acids help the body burn fat around the mid-section—basically, your waist and stomach—which is most people's trouble spot. I've often noticed that people who stick to a very low-fat diet tend to be a bit thicker around the middle, no matter how little they weigh. So always pick the full-fat version when you're choosing what to eat; choose butter over margarine and regular hummus over the so-called "diet" version. Not only will the full-fat products make you cleaner and keep you fuller for longer, but the "low-fat" options are usually pumped full of toxic, processed, low-calorie sugar, salt, and sweeteners.

*top tip

Have half an avocado on its own as a snack or with oatcakes for a delicious, filling, stress-busting breakfast.

HOLLY'S STORY

"My boyfriend Darren and I met and fell in love 12 months ago and it became our year of saying 'yes' to everything! More wine? Sure! Dessert or cheese platter... Oooh should we have both? Unsurprisingly, our middles started to grow.

We'd both struggled with fluctuating weight over the years and it caused us angst and frustration. I tried the Clean & Lean diet a couple of times but never fully committed to it. However, at the start of this year I was determined to succeed. There was no pressure for Darren to join in but within two days he'd read the book too and become the official cheerleader for Clean & Lean.

We had a couple of rough days and for me, some big confrontations about my relationship with food and alcohol. Two weeks in, we'd dropped a collective 28½ lbs, felt incredibly motivated and calm. For me, it's not just about the weight loss. Living Clean & Lean has given us energy and focus, which is critical as I run my own business. But the bigger motivation is that I met the love of my life when I was older. I want to do everything I can to ensure that our 'happily ever after' lasts a really really long time."

Most people overeat "low-fat" diet products too, because they are lulled by them into a false sense of security. When you're eating low-fat hummus, for example, it's tempting to polish off half a tub because there's a great big sticker on the packet reminding you that it's "reduced fat" or "lite." Also, low-fat products often don't contain as much flavor. For example, butter contains something called CLA which is great for fat burning, plus it enhances the flavor of food making it richer, so satisfying your appetite in a way that a low-fat spread never will. I'd much rather my clients put a little bit of organic butter on their food (which is all they need to keep their taste buds happy), rather than smothering it with a toxic, processed, low-fat spread that will never, ever satisfy them.

Good fat also helps your body to absorb vitamins and minerals better. Take a salad, for example—if you eat it on its own, you'll still get all the benefits from all those great vegetables, but it might leave you feeling a bit unsatisfied and hungry an hour or so later. But if you add some fat to it—say, half an avocado or a drizzle of olive oil—your body will be able to absorb the nutrients much better. And remember—as I explained earlier—a body full of nutrients doesn't feel hungry; it burns fat a lot quicker and it doesn't feel tired (so doesn't need to snack on toxic sugar to keep it going). Adding fat to a salad also makes it more satisfying, so you'll feel full hours after eating it and won't need to snack as much.

Another advantage of good fat is that it helps to cushion your joints from wear and tear. If you exercise, you absolutely have to have some fat in your diet to prevent injuries. It also boosts your concentration and energy levels, plus it gives you amazing hair, skin, and nails (see p. 112 to find out why a fat-free diet gives you wrinkles).

Low-fat varieties of popular foods are packed with salt and sugar—often two or three times as much as the normal version—making them LESS healthy.

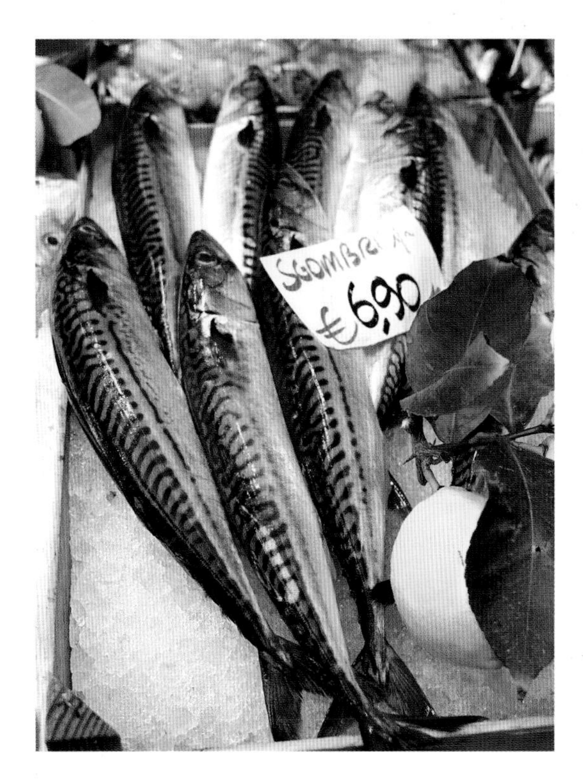

In my opinion eating enough good fat also banishes the following (all-too-common) problems:
✳ Inability to concentrate
✳ Sluggishness
✳ Feeling physically full, but still hungry (i.e. that feeling you get when you're peckish shortly after a meal)
✳ Craving something sweet after food
✳ A sudden mid-afternoon energy drop
✳ Difficulty waking up in the morning
✳ A feeling of lethargy and fatigue

HOW TO CHOOSE A SUPPLEMENT

There are so many fish oil supplements on the market—some are high quality, and some aren't. A good way of testing any kind of pill or supplement is to leave it in a glass of water overnight. A good-quality pill will break down and dissolve—a bad one won't, which implies that when you take it, it's going straight through you.

NUTS & SEEDS

✳ Almonds
✳ Pecans
✳ Walnuts
✳ Brazil nuts
✳ Pistachios
✳ Macadamias
✳ Cashews
✳ Chestnuts
✳ Sesame seeds
✳ Peanuts
✳ Sunflower seeds
✳ Pumpkin seeds
✳ Flaxseed (ground only)

FISH

The following are all rich in fatty acids, which are essential for good health
✳ Salmon*
✳ Trout
✳ Pilchards
✳ Mackerel*
✳ Anchovies
✳ Herring
✳ Sardines
✳ Kippers
✳ Whitebait
✳ Tuna* (go for fresh steaks or the kind in glass jars—these are much better for you than the canned stuff)
✳ Swordfish*
✳ Lemon sole
✳ Haddock
✳ Monkfish
✳ John Dory
✳ Red snapper
✳ Plaice
✳ Skate
✳ Halibut
✳ Dover sole
✳ Red and grey mullet
✳ Sea bass
✳ Sea bream
*These contain mercury, so limit yourself to two or three servings a week (or, if you're pregnant, just one or two servings a week)

CLEAN & LEAN OILS FOR COOKING

When cooking on low to medium heat:

* Macadamia nut oil * Avocado oil * Olive oil

When cooking on high heat:

* Ghee * Coconut oil* * Organic extra virgin

Note: Don't cook with olive oil on a high heat—cold olive oil is a healthy fat full of goodness, but, heated up, it becomes a bad fat. Olive oil breaks down at high temperatures and becomes more carcinogenic (i.e. toxic). Only ever use olive oil cold as a salad dressing or heat it up gently for short periods (say, if you're stir-frying shrimp or vegetables for a few minutes).

* Coconut oil is hugely popular amongst models thanks to its health and body-boosting benefits. The oil contains fatty acids that speed up your metabolism, and leave your hair and skin smooth and healthy. It can also withstand a high cooking temperature, unlike olive oil.

How to eat fat

For a start, you need to know the difference between good (clean) fat and bad (toxic) fat. Good fat is monounsaturated fat (MUFA), and it's found mainly in nuts, avocados, and olive oil. It helps to lower bad cholesterol and reduces overall body fat by revving up your metabolism. Then there's polyunsaturated fat, which also lowers bad cholesterol levels, and is found mainly in fish and seafood. As I've said before, a meal or snack is not complete (or healthy), unless it has a bit of fat with it, so see my Clean & Lean fat lists below.

I tell my clients to take Omega Brilliance, an omega-3 fish oil supplement too and I always say, if you don't take any other supplements, then at least take these. They top up levels of essential fatty acids and also encourage your body to burn fat (around your stomach and waist in particular), plus they boost energy levels and improve your skin. Bodyism Fish Oil sold at my gym and online has been certified to contain no toxic chemicals or additives at all. Remember, you don't need my supplements, they just accelerate the process and make things a little easier.

The following fish aren't oily or as rich in omega-3 fatty acids as those listed below, but they're still incredibly healthy. Cod is also fantastic for you, but it's massively overfished at the moment, so avoid it if you can.

Bad fats

There are a few bad types of fat that give all the other fats a bad name. Trans fats are the worst (see also p. 40) and are found in nearly all processed foods. Food manufacturers created trans fats (basically, a nasty reheated oil) to prolong their products' shelf life and add flavor. Fresh, clean, organic food goes off very quickly because it contains nothing unnatural or toxic to preserve it, but food that contains trans fats lasts for ages (think of those muffins that survive in sweaty plastic wrappers for months on end—yuck). A good rule of thumb is to only eat foods that go bad after a few days.

Trans fats are associated with some of the scariest health risks of all the fats. They've been linked to obesity, some cancers, and even infertility. People who eat trans fats have higher blood levels of interleukin-6, which, research shows, increases your risk of heart disease, and can also reduce muscle tone and metabolism.

Former Governor of California Arnold Schwarzenegger banned trans fats from all LA restaurants. They are seriously bad news—even worse than saturated fat (see below)—and you should avoid them at all costs. The worst offenders are some processed biscuits, cookies, muffins, margarines, pastries, and potato chips, but they can also be found in diet foods, mousses, protein shakes, and bars and just about anything with a long shelf life. Food manufacturers don't always list trans fats as such on their ingredients lists because they know they've got such a bad reputation; avoid "hydrogenated oil," "hydrogenated vegetable fat" and "partially hydrogenated vegetable oil," which are trans fats hiding under a different name.

Then there is saturated fat. This isn't as bad as trans fat, because it's natural. But it's still fattening, so it's best to avoid it where possible and only indulge occasionally. Often called "sat fat" on food packages, this raises bad cholesterol levels and is found mainly in animal products like meat and full-fat dairy.

WHAT'S THE DIFFERENCE BETWEEN FAT AND PROTEIN?

Protein is the building block of every hormone and increases your metabolism. Protein is basically anything that used to run, walk, swim, or fly. For example, chicken, eggs (from something that used to walk), fish, shellfish, beef etc. It's made up of amino acids, which help lay down lean muscle mass, which, as well as giving you the appearance of looking toned, also helps to speed up your metabolism and keep you strong and healthy.

Fat comes in many forms, and there are good and bad fats. The good ones are called essential fatty acids (EFAs)—they're essential because we can't produce them ourselves. Good fats give us a full feeling and are incredibly beneficial for just about every system and process within the body.

However, when you eat meat, fat is the white stuff on the edges and generally the harder the fat, the more full of toxins it is, so stay away from the hard fat on the side of meat. Stay away from trans fats—if you see trans fat on the label, put it back on the shelf.

Remember!

Try to get all your fat from food or good-quality supplements. Avoid adding it to meals in the form of margarine, mayo, or creamy sauces. If you pick foods that are rich in natural fat (such as eggs, salmon, etc.), you won't need to add more toxic fat. Keep it as clean and as natural as possible.

Here's my quick at-a-glance guide to bad fat:

Anything with a crust—next time you order a pie, take off the pastry and enjoy the filling.

Pizza—most packaged pizzas are layer upon layer of wheat (which converts to fat), topped with cheese that's processed and laced with additives. The actual topping—the chicken and mushrooms, for example—make up a tiny percentage of the whole pizza.

Prepared meals—you can find bad fat in practically every single packaged food. Just make your own meal—it takes a little longer, but it'll make you cleaner and leaner.

Olive oil—WHEN it is heated to high temperatures.

Shop-bought cakes, cookies, and muffins—despite what the labels may say, they haven't been "home-baked"—they've been processed in a factory and pumped full of junk to keep them "fresh" for as long as possible.

Anything described as deep-fried, sautéed, or breaded—for obvious reasons!

Any obvious fat on an animal product—for example, the white rind on a slice of bacon. Don't forget, toxins are stored in the fat of animals (as they are in humans), so always cut off the white, hard fat.

Salad dressings—they're usually high in sugar, salt and trans fats. Add good fat (and clean flavor) to your salad instead by ordering extra avocado or using extra-virgin olive oil. And remember, don't be fooled by a low-fat salad dressing—remember, low fat just means high in sugar, which in turn converts to fat around your waist.

What about dairy?

Almost all my clients ask me about dairy—usually along the lines of, "Will it make me fat?" or, "Will giving it up make me slim?" The answer is that dairy is OK if you're OK with it—if it doesn't make you bloated or uncomfortably full, keep having it. But many people find the lactose in cow's milk hard to digest, so if you're regularly gassy or bloated then you may be intolerant. In which case, reduce the amount you drink or eliminate it from your diet and replace it with more easily digested alternatives like almond, oat, rice, or hazelnut milk.

If you are having milk, use the best you can find. Ideally, this means raw, organic, unpasteurized and unhomogenized milk. Pasteurization involves heating

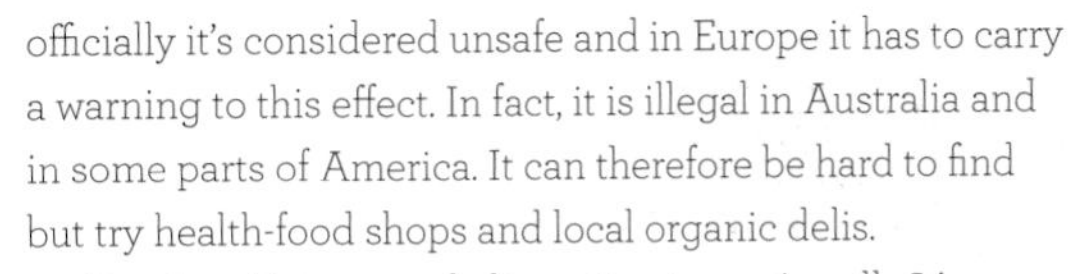

milk to just below boiling point; a process that kills bacteria but also—crucially for the food manufacturers—extends the shelf life of milk. However, the process also kills off lots of the goodness, and unpasteurized milk has much higher levels of nutrients and omega 3s. As I've been saying all along, the less a food has been tampered with, the better it is. However, unpasteurized milk is fairly controversial—officially it's considered unsafe and in Europe it has to carry a warning to this effect. In fact, it is illegal in Australia and in some parts of America. It can therefore be hard to find but try health-food shops and local organic delis.

Goat's milk is a good alternative to cow's milk. It's actually better for you because it's easier to digest, and it's closer in molecular structure to human breast milk, which your body is designed to handle.

It almost goes without saying that your milk should be organic. If you can't afford much in the way of organic food, just buy organic milk (and meat). Countless studies show that organic milk contains more nutrients than non-organic, plus it contains omega-3 fatty acids. The same goes for yogurt—forget the low-fat/high-sugar rubbish; just buy organic, full-fat goat yogurt instead.

And what about cheese?

Well, it's full of saturated fat, so it's best eaten in moderation. As a rule, if it's bright yellow and packed in slices, avoid it altogether. (Remember, look beyond those "high in calcium" claims on the packet—and a little more carefully at the ingredients. If it contains anything you can't pronounce, ditch it.) A good natural cheese, on the other hand (organic of course), can contain good nutrients and minerals. Try to buy sheep or goat cheese as these tend to be a little less processed. Once you've finished your 14-day Kickstart, you can introduce a little bit of good cheese into your diet.

How to cook fat the Clean & Lean way

Here are some tips on keeping your fat as healthy as possible when you're preparing it:

Never, ever microwave your protein. Remember, microwaves kill the goodness in food. With protein, microwaves also alter the molecular structure, leaving it unrecognisable to your gut wall. I would NEVER microwave my food.

Never overcook your meat—the longer it cooks, the more goodness is lost. (Note: always cook chicken thoroughly because it has such a high food-poisoning risk.) Never blacken or char your meat or fish—the black stuff is toxic to your system. Bake, steam, or boil (lightly)—you'll retain more of the vitamins.

BAD	BETTER	BEST
Cooking fats—even olive oil, which breaks down easily at high temperatures, making fat rancid	**Macadamia nut oil**—a great monounsaturated fat that has been shown to lower bad cholesterol	**Organic extra-virgin coconut oil**—this doesn't break down at high temperatures and tastes amazing
Store-bought salad dressing—packed with sugar and salt	**Extra-virgin olive oil**—good fats to help fill you up, making your salad a complete dish	**Organic, cold-pressed extra-virgin olive oil**—the least processed of all oils. It's got the most nutrients and the most flavor
Margarine—heavily processed and often contains artificial colorings	**Regular butter**—more natural, and has far more flavor than margarine so you won't use as much	**Unsalted grass-fed butter**—the least processed of butters
Hydrogenated/partially hydrogenated oils (trans fats)—can lead to clogging of arteries	**Vegetable oil**—has been shown to improve your metabolism	**Fats naturally found in oily fish**—salmon, mackerel, albacore tuna, herring and sardines; high in omega-3s
Packaged, pre-made guacamole—processed and packed with preservatives and E numbers; usually uses overripe avocados	**Homemade guacamole**—a better alternative and a really great dip	**Clean & Lean Guacamole**—packed with good fats, vegetables, antioxidants and flavor (see p. 97 for recipe)
Roasted and salted nuts—the roasting process can make the nuts go rancid	**Raw salted nuts**—raw nuts are high in omega 3 oils, which are degraded by heat, so they are better for you than roasted nuts	**Raw unsalted nuts**—in their most natural, least processed form; a super Clean & Lean snack
Vegetable-based margarines—soy or sunflower—highly processed and are generally highly sprayed with pesticides	**Organic cow's butter**—more natural than margarine, and because of its better flavor you'll use less	**Organic goat butter**—goat butter is high in protein and calcium, and contains higher levels of fatty acids than cow's butter, meaning many people find it easier to digest
Doughnuts—the worst of all pastries, packed with additives and sugar that destroy any attempts at fat loss	**Muffin from a health-food shop**—it may contain some fiber and fruit (and satisfy your sweet craving), but it's still pumped full of fat and sugar	**Homemade fruit and nut muffin**—the perfect mix of fat and good sugar to satisfy your sweet craving and help fill you up; eat the fat (nuts) first
Croissant or pain au chocolat (fancy name for a chocolate sausage roll)—zero-fiber, dead pastry soaked in bad fats	**Muffin from a health-food shop** (see above)	**Homemade organic oat muffin with cinnamon**—cinnamon helps regulate blood sugar levels and reduces sugar cravings

BAD	BETTER	BEST
Bacon—full of nitrates which drag nutrients from your body, including essential vitamins A, C and E	**Chicken thigh**—a good source of protein and nitrate-free	**Organic, free-range chicken breast**—super-lean and free from hormones
Potato chips—the thinner they are, the fewer nutrients and more bad fats they contain	**Salted, unroasted nuts**—a much better alternative for satisfying hunger; but one small handful, maximum!	**Raw, organic, unsalted nuts**—protein in a clean, raw form; again, keep the quantity small—one handful only
Fried chicken—usually poor-quality meat surrounded by a layer of lard	**BBQ chicken with salad**—better-quality protein and a lot less fat; just take off the skin to avoid the toxins that cause cellulite (see p. 97)	**Turkey breast and super greens**—turkey is a very lean meat that helps you sleep well
Burger and fries—usually the bread is so sugary, it's classified as a pastry; poor-quality meat and sometimes not even real potato in the fries	**Beef patty and salad**—breadless means less empty carbs and more room for the clean salad	**Lean beef stir-fry with loads of vegetables**—quick and delicious; feeds your muscles and burns fat
Deep-fried fish—clogs up your heart and causes cellulite (see p. 170)	**Pan-fried fish and salad**—if you're in a restaurant always ask for your fish to be pan fried as lots of the fat drips away	**Grilled fish and a green salad**—if you want to get rid of your cellulite have this every night; it's perfect—full of fiber and super lean
Lamb korma —swimming in cream, which is normally full of salt	**Lamb stew**—less heavy and made with vegetables to add some mineral content	**Stir-fried lamb with vegetables**—high-nutrient, low-calorie
Pizza—high in wheat and salt	**Homemade pizza**—fresh ingredients contain a higher nutrient and mineral content	**Homemade pizza with a thin, gluten-free base**
Sausage rolls—poor-quality meat wrapped in buttery pastry	**Lamb or chicken kebab with salad**—skip the unhealthy pastry and go for a better quality meat	**Organic lamb or chicken with salad**—organic meat is hormone-free and the salad is packed with nutrients
Sausage—the meat is often poor quality and high in fat	**Organic sausage**—good-quality meat	**Grass-fed organic lamb steak**—a good source of iron
Battery eggs—produced by hens housed in flocks up to 1,000 times their natural size	**Free-range eggs**—contain 15 to 30 times less cholesterol than battery eggs	**Organic eggs**—the highest bio-availability of any protein and contains all the amino acids

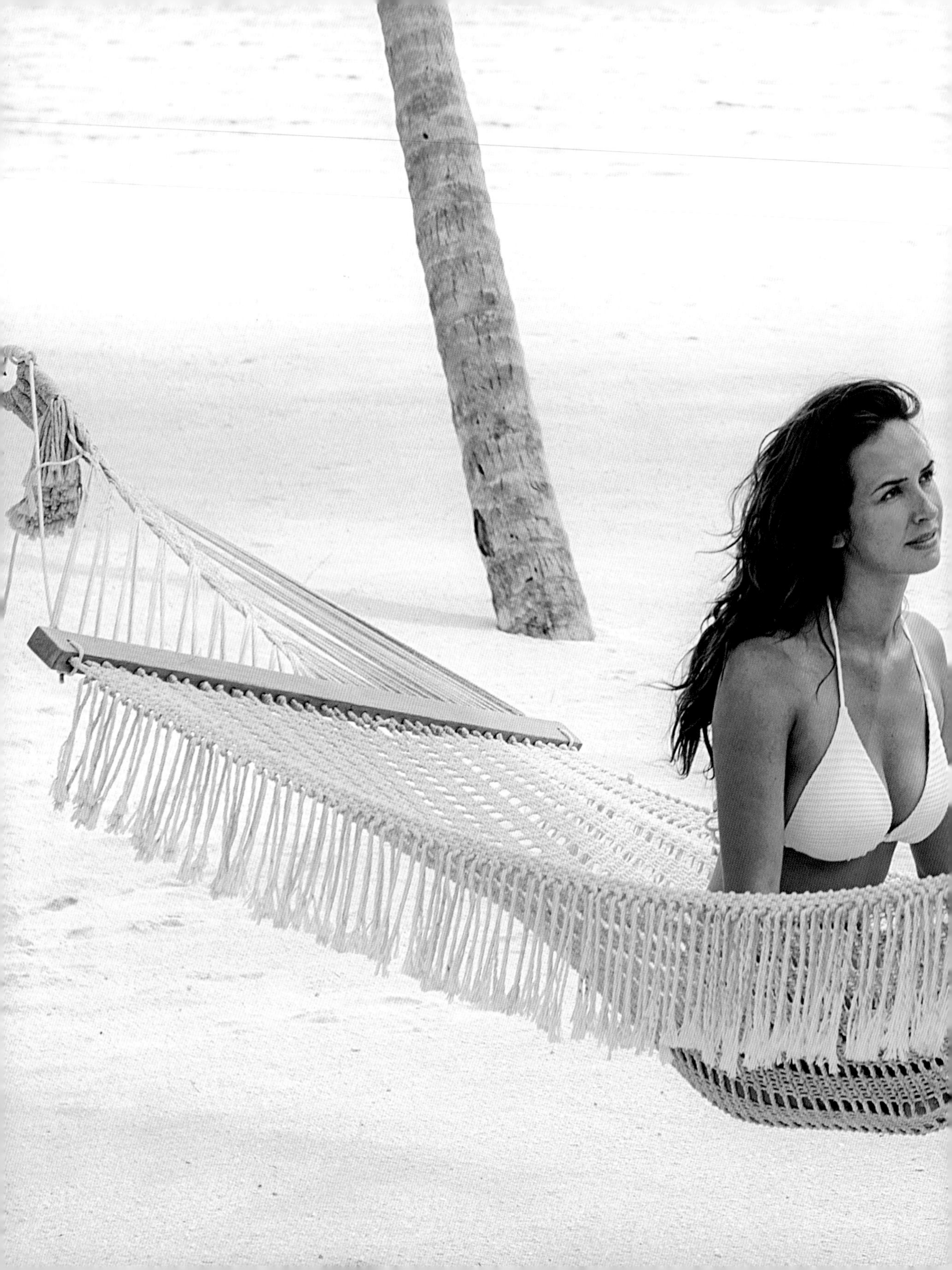

CHAPTER 6

YOUR 14-DAY KICKSTART

THIS CHAPTER WILL REVEAL...

WHY IT'S WORTH BUYING ORGANIC FOOD

WHY YOU SHOULD NEVER MICROWAVE YOUR FOOD

14 DAYS' WORTH OF EASY-TO-PREPARE MEALS

PART TWO

THE LEAN SECTION

This plan is flexible, in that you can add extra green vegetables to a meal if you're still hungry, and feel free to mix and match the days. For example, something like grilled sea bass is easier to cook for lunch on the weekend, rather than during the week, if you work in an office. For that reason, it's best to start the plan on the weekend when you'll have more time to prepare the meals. You'll need recipes for some of the meals (for these and more Clean & Lean recipes, see Chapter 7). In fact, if you don't like the look of some of the suggestions here you can always substitute meal suggestions from the recipes in Chapter 7.

Why it's worth buying organic food

If possible, try to buy everything organic. This is especially important when it comes to vegetables, dairy, eggs, and meat. If you do buy non-organic chicken, always remove the skin because that's where many of the toxins are stored. And try to serve vegetables as raw as possible, and where you do cook them make sure you grill, steam, sauté, or stir-fry them, rather than frying, boiling, or microwaving.

Why you shouldn't microwave your food

The reason for this is quite simple: because it seems far more natural to just heat food on something hot. Where possible, always heat food through in a pan instead of using the microwave.

OPTIONS

There are plenty of non-meat options for vegetarians in the Clean & Lean plan. Just substitute the vegetarian options accordingly.

BEST WAYS:

Steaming
Steaming is one of the healthiest ways to cook fish, meat and vegetables as it retains nearly all the nutrients (and flavor) and doesn't add any fat.

Blanching
This is a way of cooking vegetables that keeps them crisp and tender, while retaining lots of the nutrients. You boil them for a short amount of time, so that they're barely cooked, then you remove them from the heat, drain, then add them to a bowl of icy water. Wait until they're no longer warm, then quickly reheat them (boil/steam/grill for 30 seconds–1 minute).

Broiling
This is a great way of cooking meat and fish. Lots of the fat drips away, plus it gives a lovely flavor to your food.

Baking/roasting
There isn't any real difference between these two. They're methods of cooking meat, fish or vegetables using dry heat (your oven) which browns the food's exterior and cooks the middle.

WORST WAYS:

Frying
Usually, this involves cooking foods with oil in a hot pan. Firstly, the oil soaks into the food, and secondly, because that fat is heated up it becomes less healthy (cold olive oil is far healthier than hot olive oil).

Boiling
When you boil vegetables they lose many of their health-boosting nutrients. Blanching (see left) is OK because you're only boiling them for a short amount of time. But when you just boil your vegetables—for a long time—too many nutrients are lost.

Microwaving
This method may save you time, but microwaving your food is one of the worst ways to cook. Some studies have found that it can destroy up to 97 percent of the health-boosting antioxidants found in vegetables, so it's not a method of cooking I recommend.

WHAT ABOUT FRUIT?

My 14-day Clean & Lean Kickstart is low in fruit (although high in vegetables). This is because fruit contains so much sugar, and for this initial kickstart, I want to limit sugar intake as much as possible. Once you have done your first two weeks, you can reintroduce berries (raspberries, blueberries, strawberries). They're jam-packed with antioxidants and have a highly beneficial compound called proanthocyanidins which protects you against degenerative diseases, such as cancer, heart disease, and diabetes. A 2012 study from Harvard Medical even found they can reduce memory decline in old age and a 2010 study from Ohio State University found they can reduce your risk of certain cancers. In Chapter 10 I'll talk more about reintroducing other foods and drinks after the kickstart, such as coffee and wine.

*top tip

Eat local, eat fresh —find out what's in season —source local produce: farmers' markets are a great way to buy fresh, organic food and support the farmers in your community.

*top tip

Grow your own herbs and veggies: if you haven't got the space, join a community garden. Gardening is great way to move your body and you get to go home with a basket full of home grown fruit and veggies.

14-DAY KICKSTART

When you feel ready to start, follow this two-week plan. It's best to start on a weekend, when you have more time to get everything ready. Plus you won't feel so stressed or rushed, which will mean you'll be less likely to supplement the plan with a mid-afternoon chocolate bar.

We do recommend that you try out a few of our Clean & Lean shakes and products. You do NOT need to buy them, but they are there to make things easier and to accelerate the process.

Upon awakening, we recommend you try Body Brilliance with Ultimate Clean & Lean Beauty Food. After lunch, you could take one Omega Brilliance and one Multi Optimum and, before bed, Body Serenity with Ultimate Clean & Lean. Please don't feel you have to buy them, you don't. We love them and so do our clients but Clean & Lean will work without them as well. There's no hard sell here, but they are available at bodyism.com and cleanandlean.com.

DAY 1

Breakfast: Poached Eggs with Broccoli, Arugula, Grilled Tomato, and Parmesan (p. 84)

Snack: a handful of walnuts

Lunch: Clean & Lean Super Salad with Smoked Salmon (p. 98)

Snack: a handful of blueberries

Dinner: Marinated Grilled Chicken (p. 92)

DAY 2

Breakfast: Clean & Lean Super Breakfast (p. 87)

Snack: a handful of pecans

Lunch: Grilled Chicken Breast with Spicy Salsa and Spinach and Avocado Salad (p. 94)

Snack: a handful of raspberries

Dinner: Super Ground Beef Sauce (p. 111)

DAY 3

Breakfast: Toasted Rye Bread with Cinnamon Honey Butter (p. 84)

Snack: a handful of Brazil nuts

Lunch: Green Bean and Tomato Salad with Turkey (p. 107)

Snack: a handful of strawberries

Dinner: Red and Yellow Pepper Spelt Salad (p. 104)

WHAT DOES ¼ LB LOOK LIKE?

If you don't have scales to measure out your protein portion, here's a rough guide to the measurements given in the 14-day diet plan:

* **¼ lb smoked salmon** = the size of your outstretched hand (including fingers)
* **¼ lb chicken** = two thirds of the size of a regular breast
* **¼ lb beef fillet** = the size of a small hamburger

MEAL PLANNER

DAY 4

Breakfast: Poached Eggs with Broccoli, Arugula, Grilled Tomato, and Parmesan (p. 84)

Snack: a handful of mixed seeds

Lunch: Spicy Beet and Lamb Salad (p. 104)

Snack: a handful of blackberries

Dinner: Chicken, Asparagus and Cashew Nut Stir-fry (p. 111)

DAY 5

Breakfast: Clean & Lean Super Breakfast (p. 87)

Snack: a handful of cashews

Lunch: Quinoa and Roasted Pepper Salad with Seeds (p. 101)

Snack: a handful of mixed berries

Dinner: Salad of Wild Rice, Mackerel, Spiced Pecans, and Avocado (p. 102)

DAY 6

Breakfast: Fruity Clean & Lean Quinoa (p. 88)

Snack: a handful of pistachio nuts

Lunch: Cold Lamb Salad (p. 98)

Snack: a handful of blueberries

Dinner: Thai Chicken Satay (p. 93)

*top tip

Every day, upon awakening, always drink 1 glass of water with a fresh squeeze of lemon or lime and a pinch of Himalayan salt.

DAY 7

Breakfast: Poached Eggs with Broccoli, Arugula, Grilled Tomato, and Parmesan (p. 84)

Snack: a handful of almonds

Lunch: Fava Bean, Spinach and Turkey Salad (p. 107)

Snack: a handful of strawberries

Dinner: Salmon en Papillote with Ginger and Lime (p. 112)

DAY 8

Breakfast: Clean & Lean Super Breakfast (p. 87)

Snack: a handful of pecans

Lunch: Spicy Beet and Lamb Salad (p. 104)

Snack: a handful of mixed berries

Dinner: Quinoa and Roasted Pepper Salad with Seeds (p. 101)

DAY 9

Breakfast: Fruity Clean & Lean Quinoa (p. 88)

Snack: a handful of almonds

Lunch: Green Bean and Tomato Salad with Turkey (p. 107)

Snack: a handful of strawberries

Dinner: Salmon en Papillote with Ginger and Lime (p. 112)

DAY 10

Breakfast: Quick Scrambled Eggs (p. 88)

Snack: a handful of mixed seeds

Lunch: Clean & Lean Super Salad with Smoked Salmon (p. 98)

Snack: a handful of blueberries

Dinner: Grilled Chicken Breast with Spicy Salsa and Spinach and Avocado Salad (p. 94)

Food is one of our main life sources. It nourishes us, keeps us strong, and can make us look and feel amazing. It lifts our mood and our energy levels. When you view it in this way, and eat foods that are good for you, the weight will drop off.

DAY 11

Breakfast: Clean & Lean Super Breakfast (p. 87)

Snack: a handful of brazil nuts

Lunch: Elle's Kale, Sprout, and Goat Cheese Salad (p. 94)

Snack: a handful of raspberries

Dinner: Spicy Beet and Lamb Salad (p. 104)

DAY 12

Breakfast: Easy Eggs Florentine with Goat Cheese (p. 91)

Snack: a handful of cashews

Lunch: Cold Lamb Salad (p. 98)

Snack: a handful of blackberries

Dinner: Super Ground Beef Sauce (p. 111)

DAY 13

Breakfast: Haddock, Eggs, and Peppers on Rye (p. 91)

Snack: a handful of walnuts

Lunch: Salad of Wild Rice, Mackerel, Spiced Pecans, and Avocado (p. 102)

Snack: a handful of mixed berries

Dinner: Chicken, Asparagus and Cashew Nut Stir-fry (p. 111)

DAY 14

Breakfast: Poached Eggs with Broccoli, Arugula, Grilled Tomato, and Parmesan (p. 84)

Snack: a handful of mixed nuts

Lunch: Fava Bean, Spinach and Turkey Salad (p. 107)

Snack: a handful of blueberries

Dinner: Salmon en Papillote with Ginger and Lime (p. 112)

*top tip

Every day, upon awakening, drink 1 glass of water with a fresh squeeze of lemon or lime and a pinch of Himalayan salt.

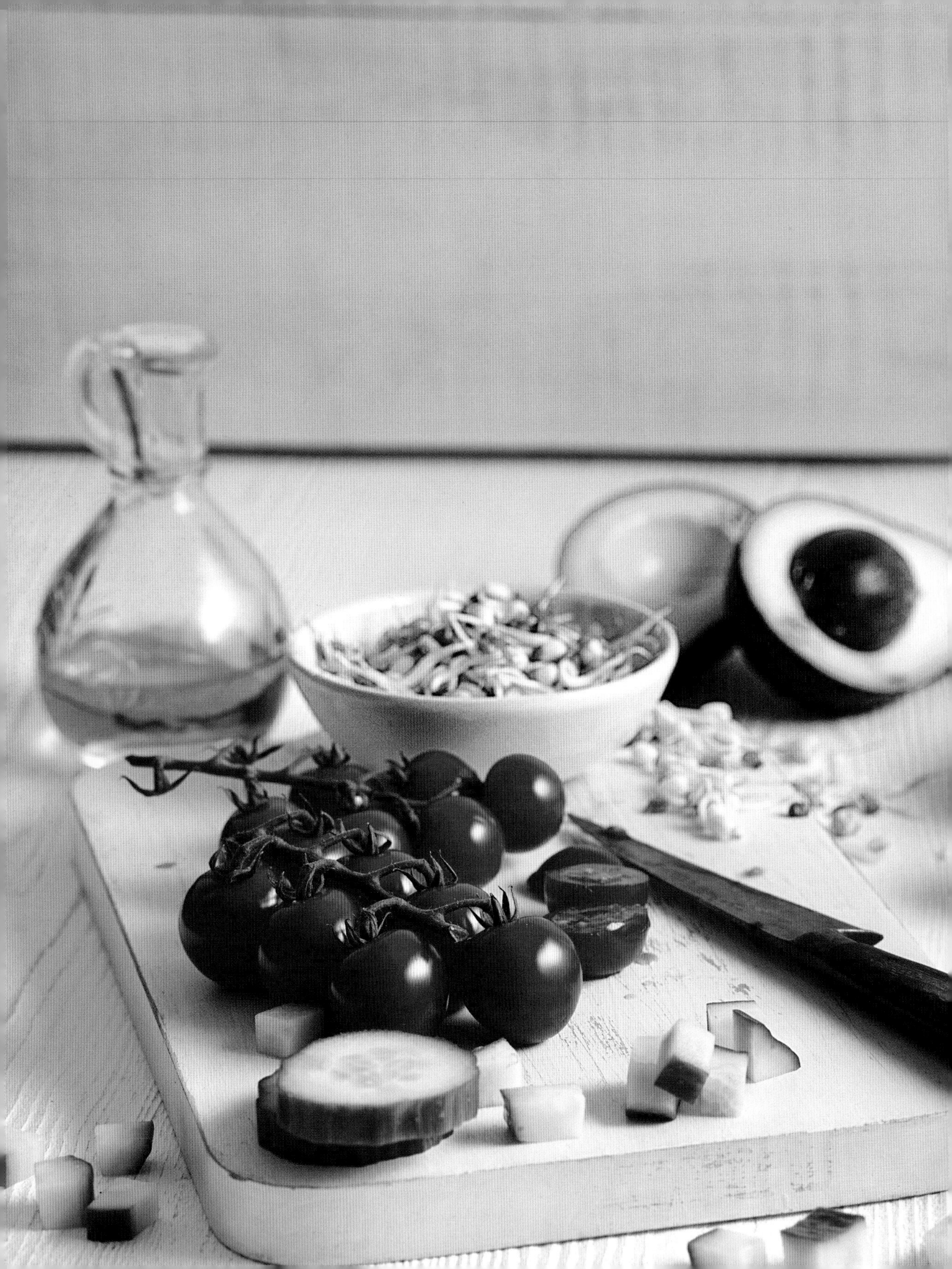

CHAPTER 7

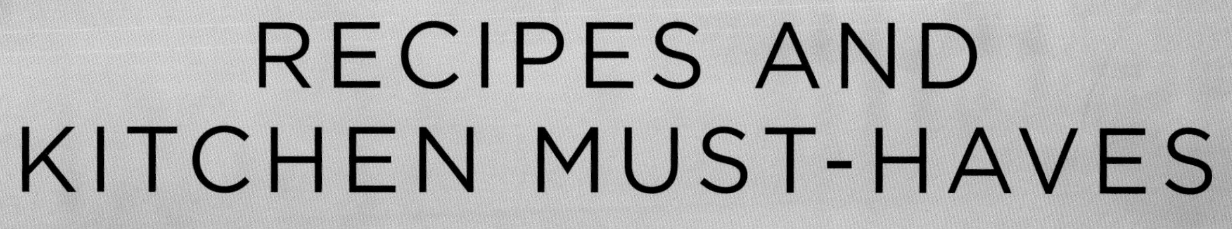

RECIPES AND KITCHEN MUST-HAVES

THIS CHAPTER WILL REVEAL…

HOW EASY IT IS TO MAKE HEALTHY MEALS

FOODS YOU SHOULD ALWAYS HAVE IN YOUR KITCHEN

THE SMOOTHIE THAT BLASTS FAT

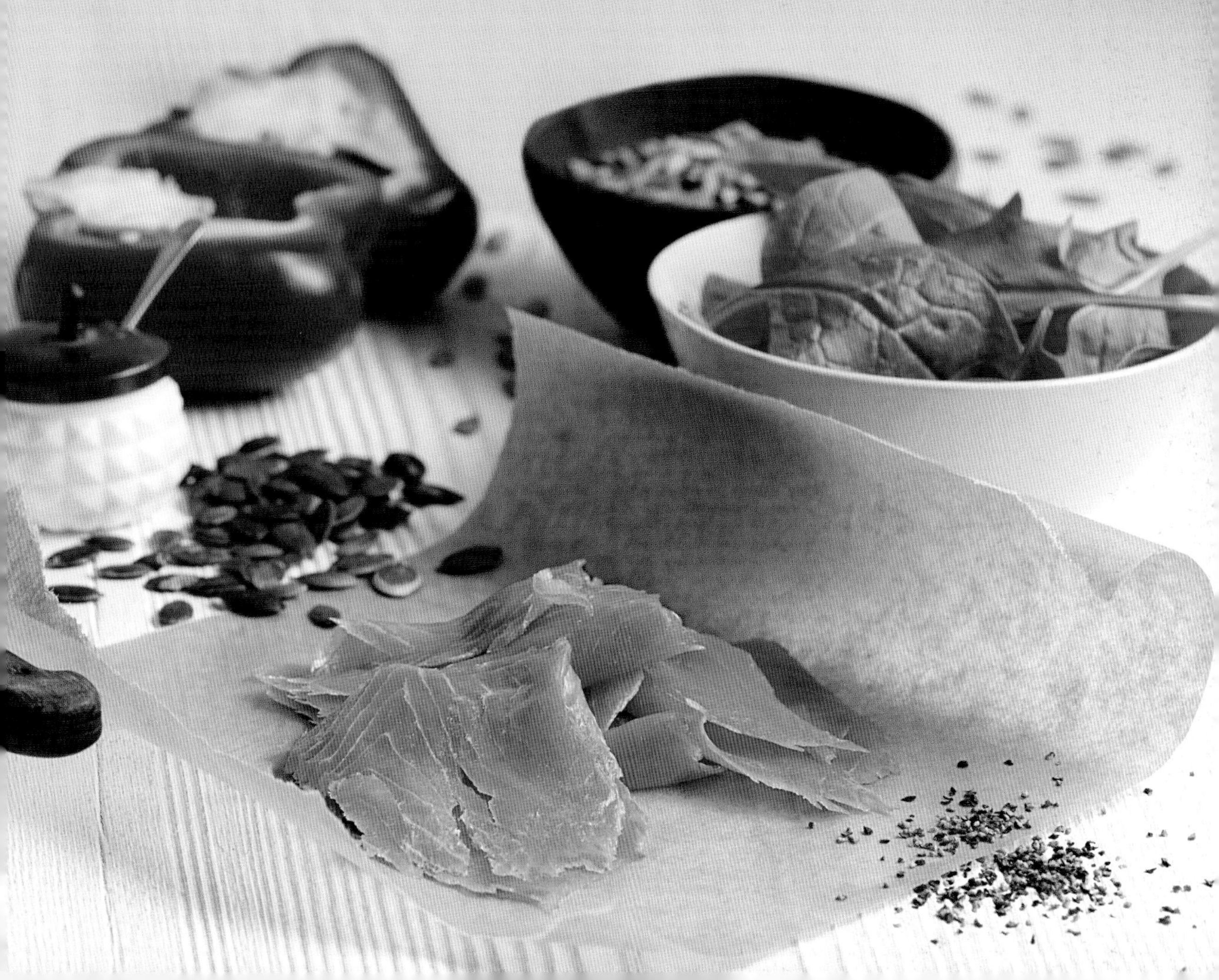

CLEAN & LEAN PROTEINS

(In no particular order)

* Chicken
* Turkey
* Lamb
* Beef
* Duck
* Liver
* All fish and shellfish (to avoid mercury, no more than two or three servings of tuna and swordfish a week)

CLEAN & LEAN VEGETABLES

* **Broccoli**—packed with vitamin C to improve immunity and magnesium and calcium, which lowers blood pressure
* **Spinach**—a good source of vitamin C, it also contains a carotenoid (a health-boosting pigment found in plant based foods), which protects against prostate and ovarian cancer
* **Asparagus**—full of vitamin B, it can help prevent memory decline as we age
* **Green beans**—one of the highest sources of dietary fiber
* **Snow peas**—a good source of vitamin C and B
* **Kale**—high in iron, this helps cell growth, liver function, and energy
* **Arugula**—a good source of vitamin A, which prevents certain cancers
* **Watercress**—another good source of vitamin A
* **Brussels sprouts**—a very good source of fiber, they also contain carotenoids that can protect against most cancers.
* **Cucumber** —they're 96 per cent water so a good source of hydration plus potassium, which boosts heart health
* **Zucchini**—another good source of fiber, plus it contains some omega 3 fatty acid which is good for heart health and metabolism
* **Avocado**—it helps your body absorb nutrients from other vegetables more efficiently so it's a good addition to salads

CLEAN & LEAN NUTS & SEEDS

* **Almonds**—they're a good source of monounsaturated fat, which improves heart health
* **Pecans**—full of fiber and vitamin E, which helps lower bad cholesterol levels
* **Walnuts**—a study from Marshall University School of Medicine in West Virginia found they contain antioxidants that can protect you from breast cancer
* **Brazil nuts**—rich in monounsaturated fats and selenium
* **Pistachios**—they contain antioxidants that lower levels of bad cholesterol
* **Macadamia nuts**—a good source of vitamin B, they can boost energy levels and decrease stress
* **Cashews**—a good source of heart-protecting antioxidants, they also contain fewer calories than most other nuts
* **Chestnuts**—they're full of fiber and a fatty acid called linoleic acid, which keeps the heart healthy
* **Sesame seeds**—these are a good source of copper that can help reduce your arthritis risk
* **Peanuts**—a good source of the antioxidant resveratrol, which is also found in the skin of red grapes and keeps the heart healthy
* **Sunflower seeds**—a great source of vitamin E that keeps the skin smooth and plump and brain cells healthy
* **Pumpkin seeds**—full of zinc, which can improve sleep and immunity, plus they can also help men's fertility
* **Flax seeds**—(ground only) because if you don't grind them they can get stuck in your intestine and go rancid and rotten... so grind them up! They're great for an essential fatty acid and fiber boost
* **Chia seeds**—nutrient-dense source of protein and essential fatty acids

CLEAN & LEAN FLAVORS

* Extra-virgin olive oil for dressings (the best you can buy)
* Walnut oil
* White wine vinegar
* Sesame oil
* Light olive oil (for cooking)
* Basil-infused olive oil
* Garlic-infused olive oil
* Flaxseed oil
* Tamari soy sauce (gluten free)
* Good-quality mayonnaise
* Dijon mustard
* Lemons
* Limes
* Cilantro
* Dill
* Parsley
* Thyme
* Chile
* Cinnamon
* Garlic
* Ginger

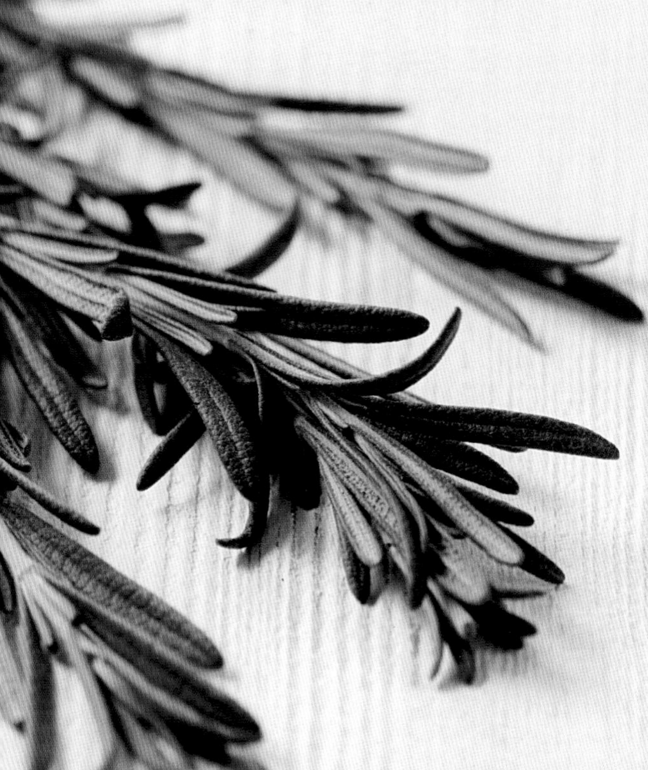

James' top ten foods

Cinnamon First of all, cinnamon's most amazing property is that it can regulate blood-sugar levels (therefore hunger and cravings) and bad cholesterol. It's also an anti-inflammatory so it can help with aches and pains. I sprinkle it in my coffee.

Garlic This helps with so many things, the list is almost too long. But here's a start: it's antiviral, an antioxidant, and helps lower bad cholesterol. Garlic is also a great tool for weight loss. The most effective way to eat it is by crushing it—the more finely crushed the better, as it releases two fat-burning enzymes. So get into garlic! Cook with it and if you're really hardcore, chew that sucker!

Blueberries These are good for snacking on—loaded with disease-fighting antioxidants, as well as anti-cancer properties.

Eggs Eggs help you build muscle because they're such a great source of protein. They also help you stay fuller for longer, and several studies show that people who have eggs for breakfast tend to be slimmer and have fewer sugar cravings. Most of the nutrients are found in the yolk, including vitamin B12, which helps the body metabolize fat, so don't be tempted to have an egg-white omelette.

Avocado A great monounsaturated fat that has been shown to lower cholesterol and helps your body work off belly fat. I have one most days with breakfast.

Coconut oil The health benefits of coconut oil are phenomenal, and many supermodels drink a teaspoon every day. It helps with weight loss, it can ease digestive problems such as bloating, it strengthens your immunity, and it keeps your cholesterol levels healthy. You can cook with it (it's one of the few oils that retains its health benefits when heated). Pour it over just about anything, from salads to poached eggs to grilled vegetables.

Good-quality coffee Full of antioxidants, plus it helps to burn fat when drunk before exercise. I stick to one a day, though.

Wild salmon The omega-3 fatty acids in oily fish like salmon, tuna, and trout help to burn belly fat and speed up a slow metabolism.

Broccoli This truly deserves the name "superfood"—loaded with nutrients and health benefits.

Spinach Full of iron, which boosts your energy levels and increases muscle endurance.

BREAKFASTS

Toasted Rye Bread with Cinnamon Honey Butter

Serves 2

Ingredients

7 tablespoons organic unsalted butter
2 tablespoons Manuka honey
½ teaspoon ground cinnamon
4 slices rye bread
2 handfuls of almonds

Method

1 Beat together the butter, honey, and cinnamon until light and fluffy. Chill in the refrigerator until set.

2 Toast the rye bread and spread with the cinnamon butter. Scatter with the almonds and serve.

Poached Eggs with Broccoli, Arugula, Broiled Tomato, and Parmesan

Serves 4

Ingredients

2 tomatoes, halved
1 broccoli, cut into florets
4 fresh organic eggs
Parmesan, for sprinkling
arugula, to serve

Method

1 Heat the broiler to high and place the tomatoes under it for a few minutes until colored.

2 While the tomatoes are cooking, steam the broccoli for 3–4 minutes until just tender, then set aside.

3 Meanwhile, bring a pan of water to a boil. Stir the water rapidly to create a whirlpool, and crack the first egg into the center; the swirling water should bring the egg together. Repeat with the remaining eggs (3–4 minutes is sufficient cooking time).

4 Serve each egg with the broccoli and broiled tomato. Grate a little Parmesan over the top, and scatter arugula over the plate.

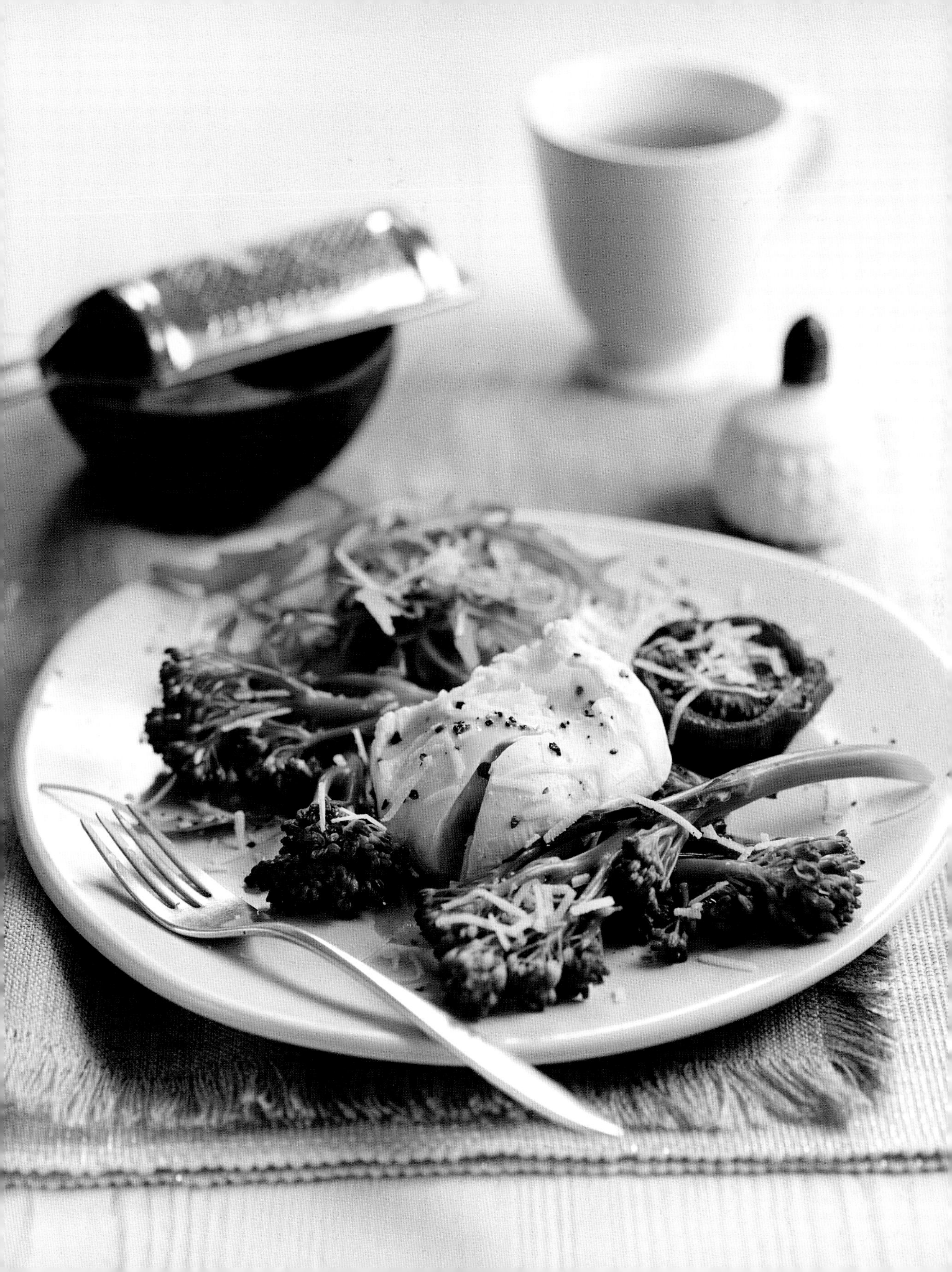

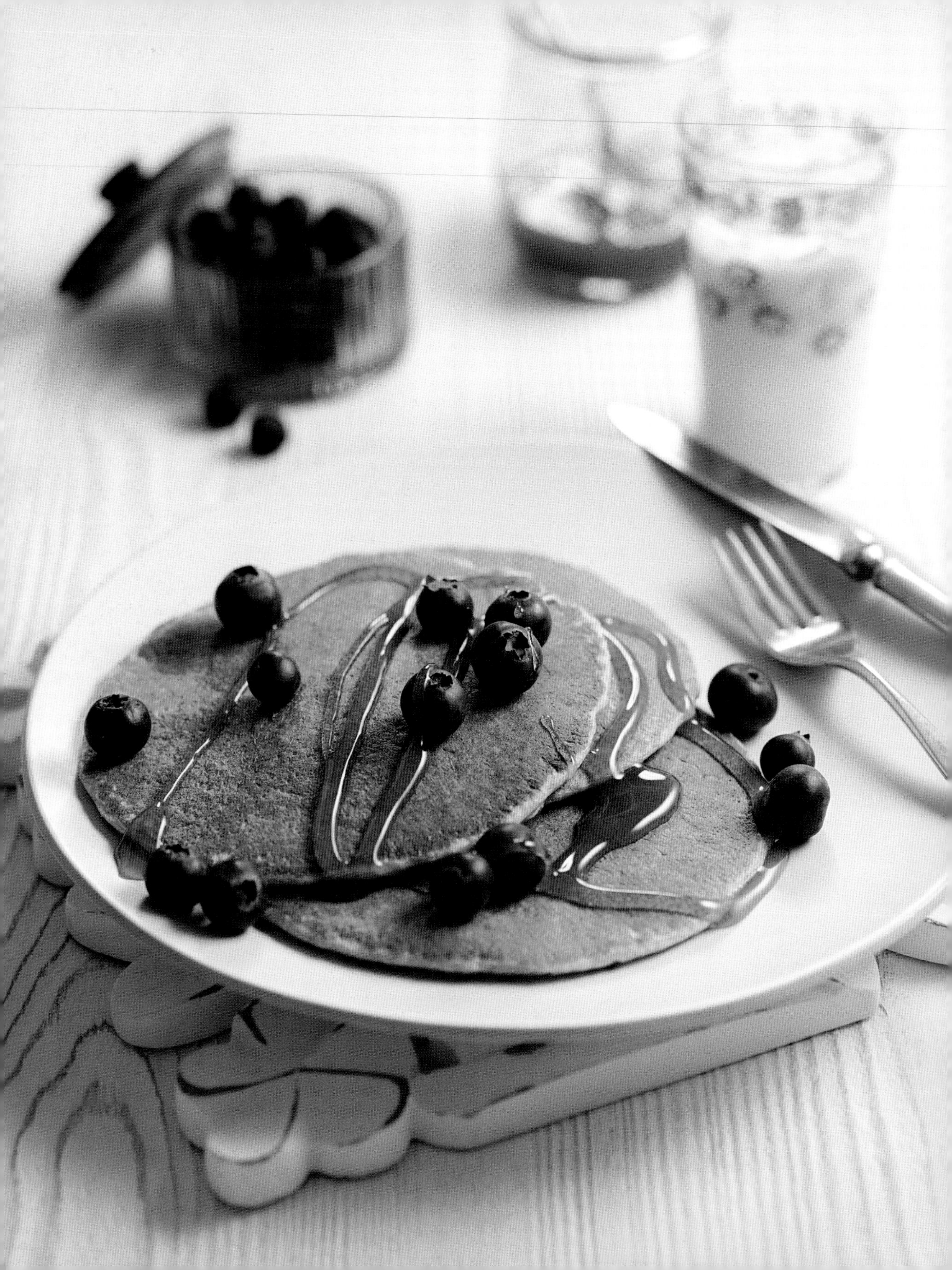

Clean & Lean Pancakes

Serves 2–4

Ingredients

⅔ cup organic rolled oats
1 cup ricotta or cottage cheese
4 eggs
1 teaspoon ground cinnamon
1 cup blueberries
2 tablespoons plain yogurt

Method

1 Blend the oats, cheese, eggs and cinnamon in a food processor until you have a smooth batter.

2 Heat a nonstick, heavy-bottomed frying pan, then pour in ladlefuls of batter and cook for 2–3 minutes on each side.

3 Serve warm, with the blueberries and yogurt.

Clean & Lean Super Breakfast

Serves 1

Ingredients

2 tablespoons oats
2 Brazil nuts
2 almonds
2 walnuts or pecans
1 teaspoon ground flaxseed
1 tablespoon pumpkin seeds
1 teaspoon chia seeds
¼ cup rice milk
¼ cup filtered water

Method

1 Soak the oats, nuts, and seeds in the rice milk and water, and refrigerate overnight.

2 In the morning, process in a blender until smooth, then drink immediately.

*it's easy

Always eat within an hour of waking up; otherwise your body will become stressed.

Quick Scrambled Eggs

Serves 1

Ingredients

2 organic eggs
generous pinch of sea salt and freshly ground black pepper
splash of milk
½ tablespoon unsalted butter
large handful of spinach
½ avocado, sliced
1 scallion, chopped
a sprinkling of cayenne pepper

Method

1 Break the eggs into a bowl, season, and whisk together with a splash of milk.

2 Melt the butter in a saucepan and then add the egg mixture, stirring all the time until they are scrambled and cooked to your liking. Just before they are ready, stir in the spinach so that it wilts slightly.

3 Serve the eggs on a plate with the avocado. Scatter the scallions over the top, and add a sprinkling of cayenne pepper to taste.

Fruity Clean & Lean Quinoa

Serves 2

Ingredients

1 cup almond or rice milk
¼ cup quinoa
⅓ cup blackberries
⅓ cup blueberries
1 tablespoon chopped pecans
Greek yogurt, to serve

Method

1 In a small saucepan, bring the almond or rice milk to a boil. Stir in the quinoa, reduce the heat to low, and simmer gently for 10 minutes or until most of the liquid has been absorbed.

2 Remove from the heat and stir in the blackberries, blueberries, and pecans. Spoon into 2 bowls and serve with Greek yogurt.

*top tip

This is bursting with nutrients and goodness with a perfect balance of carbohydrates, fats, and protein. It's particularly good for your digestion.

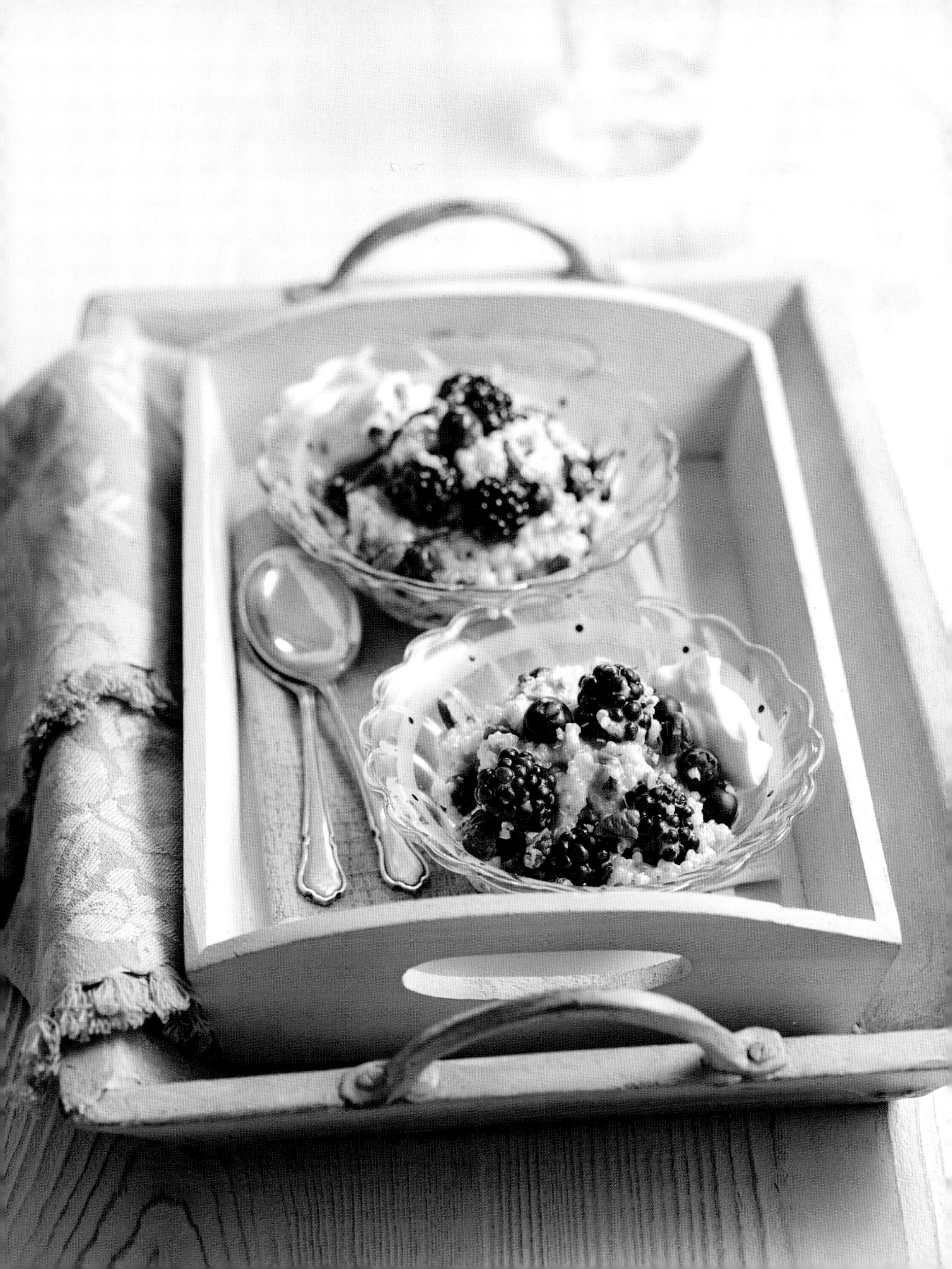

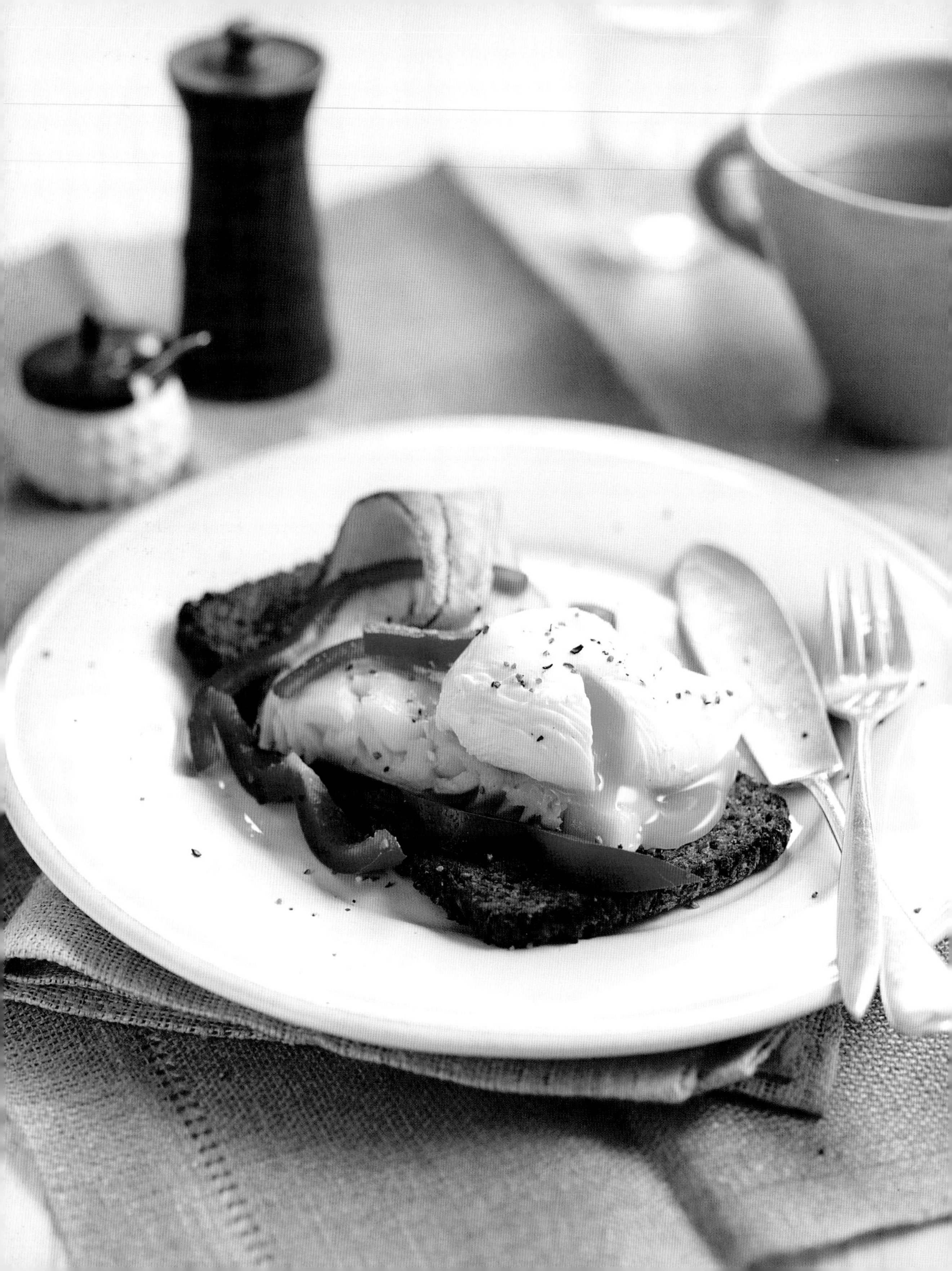

James's Favorite Breakfast—Haddock, Eggs, and Peppers on Rye

Serves 1

Ingredients

1 x 7-ounce fillet undyed smoked haddock or whitefish
2 organic eggs
½ red pepper, sliced
2 slices rye bread, toasted if you like
sea salt and freshly ground black pepper

Method

1 Heat a frying pan of water until boiling. Add the haddock fillet, cover with a lid, then turn off the heat and leave for 5 minutes.

2 Poach the eggs in a separate pan in simmering water for about 4 minutes or until the white is set but the yolk is still soft.

3 To serve, divide the haddock between the rye bread slices. Top each with a poached egg and sliced pepper, and season to taste.

Easy Egg Florentine with Goat Cheese

Serves 1

Ingredients

organic butter
2 large handfuls of fresh spinach
sea salt and freshly ground black pepper
2 organic eggs
1 tablespoon organic heavy cream
¼ cup goat cheese, crumbled

Method

1 Preheat the oven to 350°F. Lightly grease a large ramekin with butter.

2 Steam the spinach for 2 minutes until just wilted. Then season with salt and pepper, and spoon into the base of the ramekin, making a slight well in the center.

3 Break 2 organic eggs into the dish, dot with a little butter, pour in the cream, and sprinkle with the goat cheese.

4 Bake in the oven for 10 minutes until the whites are set.

*top tip

Eggs are almost the perfect food, full of a satisfying, energy-improving mix of selenium, amino acids, protein, and vitamins. Have them for breakfast to fire you up.

LUNCHES & DINNERS

Bombay Chicken Wings

Serves 6–8 as an appetizer

Ingredients

1 teaspoon curry powder
½ teaspoon ground turmeric
2 tablespoons vegetable oil
2 tablespoons finely sliced scallions
2 cloves garlic, crushed
freshly ground black pepper
15–20 organic chicken wings
cilantro leaves, to garnish

For the dipping sauce

½ cup plain yogurt
1 tablespoon chopped cilantro
1 tablespoon finely sliced scallion
¼ teaspoon hot chile sauce or oil
sea salt

Method

1 To make the dipping sauce, combine all the ingredients in a bowl; cover and refrigerate until needed.

2 In a large bowl, mix together the remaining ingredients (except the chicken wings and cilantro). Add the chicken wings, making sure all pieces are coated well. Cover the bowl with plastic wrap and refrigerate for at least 1 hour.

3 Preheat the oven to 375°F. Put the chicken wings in a baking dish and bake for 25 minutes or until golden brown. Serve with the dipping sauce and garnish with the cilantro leaves.

Marinated Grilled Chicken

Serves 4

Ingredients

6 tablespoons olive oil
¼ teaspoon Dijon mustard
1 teaspoon sea salt
½ teaspoon black pepper
1 clove garlic
zest of 1 lemon
1 tablespoon chopped chives
4 skinless organic chicken breasts, quartered
2½ cups (2 ounces) arugula
1 small red onion, finely sliced

Method

1 Pour 2 tablespoons of the olive oil into a blender, add the mustard and a ¼ teaspoon each of the salt and pepper, and process for 15 seconds. With the blender running, add another 2 tablespoons of the olive oil and process for 10 seconds. Add the remaining olive oil, plus the garlic, lemon zest, and chives, and process for 15 seconds.

2 Cover the chicken pieces in the sauce. Marinate in the fridge for at least 4 hours (or ideally overnight).

3 Preheat a broiler until hot. Put the chicken on a baking sheet, sprinkle with the remaining sea salt and pepper, then place under the broiler, about 8 inches from the heat. Broil for about 20 minutes, turning and basting with the sauce halfway through, until a fork can be inserted in the chicken with ease and it is piping hot throughout.

4 Serve with a salad of arugula and sliced red onion.

Thai Chicken Satay

Serves 4

Ingredients

1 large organic chicken breast
2 tablespoons nam pla (fish sauce)
1 tablespoon safflower oil
1 tablespoon lime juice
1 tablespoon chopped cilantro leaves
1 large clove garlic, crushed
¼ teaspoon ground cumin
1 stalk lemongrass, crushed or 1 teaspoon lemon zest

For the satay sauce

1 tablespoon safflower oil
½ red onion, chopped
1 clove garlic, crushed
1 stalk lemongrass
2 tablespoons unsalted peanuts
¾ cup low-fat coconut milk
1 teaspoon ground cumin
1 tablespoon Manuka honey
2 tablespoons fresh lime juice
¼ teaspoon sea salt
1 tablespoon soy sauce
½ teaspoon Asian hot chile sauce or oil
4 long bamboo skewers

Method

1 Place the chicken between two sheets of plastic wrap and pound gently with a rolling pin to flatten slightly. Cut the chicken into diagonal strips about ½ inch thick and thread onto 4 bamboo skewers.

2 In a shallow bowl, mix together the fish sauce, oil, lime juice, cilantro, garlic, cumin, and lemongrass. Dip each skewer into the mixture, coating well. Place the chicken in a dish, cover with plastic wrap, and refrigerate for at least 2 hours (or ideally overnight).

3 To make the satay sauce, heat the oil in a small pan, add the onion, garlic, and lemongrass, and cook, stirring, for about 3 minutes, then remove from the heat. In a food processor, chop the peanuts, then add the onion mixture, coconut milk, cumin, honey, lime juice, salt, soy sauce, and hot chile sauce or oil, and process until smooth.

4 Preheat a broiler until hot. Place the skewers on a baking sheet, and broil for 3–4 minutes on each side or until the chicken is cooked. Serve with Spicy Peanut Sauce.

Chicken Pesto with Romaine Salad

Serves 2

2 skinless, organic chicken breasts
2 teaspoons pesto
freshly ground black pepper
1 head romaine lettuce
½ red onion, sliced
1 tablespoon extra virgin olive oil
1 teaspoon lemon juice

Method

1 Preheat the oven to 375°F.

2 Make a slit in each chicken breast with a knife and put a teaspoon of pesto into each cavity. Season with black pepper and bake for 25 minutes.

3 Tear the lettuce into bite-size pieces and arrange on two plates with the onion. When ready to serve, whisk together the olive oil and lemon juice and drizzle over the lettuce. Serve the chicken alongside.

Elle's Kale, Sprout, and Goat Cheese Salad

Serves 2

Ingredients

1 bowlful kale
1 handful alfalfa sprouts
sprinkle of goat cheese
sprinkle of sunflower and pumpkin seeds
½ avocado
2 radishes, thinly sliced
sea salt and pepper, to taste
juice of ½ lemon
2 tablespoons olive oil

Method

Put the kale, alfalfa sprouts, goat cheese, seeds, avocado, and radishes in a bowl and mix. Season to taste, then dress with the lemon juice and olive oil.

*top tip

All green vegetables are all good for you, but as a general rule, the darker the better. Kale and spinach are both Clean & Lean super-ingredients.

Broiled Chicken Breasts with Spicy Salsa and Spinach and Avocado Salad

Serves 4

Ingredients

4 tablespoons fresh lime juice
¼ cup olive oil
½ teaspoon red pepper flakes
freshly ground black pepper
4 skinless organic chicken breasts
7 ounces baby spinach leaves
1 ripe avocado, peeled and sliced
1 tablespoon extra virgin olive oil
1 teaspoon lemon juice
2 tablespoons chopped cilantro leaves

For the salsa

½ red onion, finely chopped
1 tomato, finely chopped
1 tablespoon fresh lime juice
1 large clove of garlic, crushed
2 teaspoons seeded and finely sliced jalapeño pepper
¼ teaspoon ground cumin
½ teaspoon sea salt

Method

1 First make the salsa. In a bowl, mix together the onion, tomato, lime juice, garlic, jalapeño pepper, cumin, and salt. Let it sit at room temperature for about 1 hour to allow the flavors to mingle.

2 In a shallow dish, mix together the lime juice, olive oil, red pepper flakes, and pepper. Dip the chicken in the mixture until well coated. Marinate in the refrigerator for at least 1 hour.

3 Put the chicken on a baking sheet and place under a preheated broiler, 8 inches from the heat. Broil for about 8 minutes on each side, or until a fork can be inserted in the chicken with ease and the juices run clear, not pink.

4 Divide the spinach leaves and avocado slices between 4 plates. Whisk together the olive oil and lemon juice, season with salt and pepper, and drizzle over the salad. Place the chicken on top, spoon over the salsa, garnish with chopped cilantro, and serve immediately.

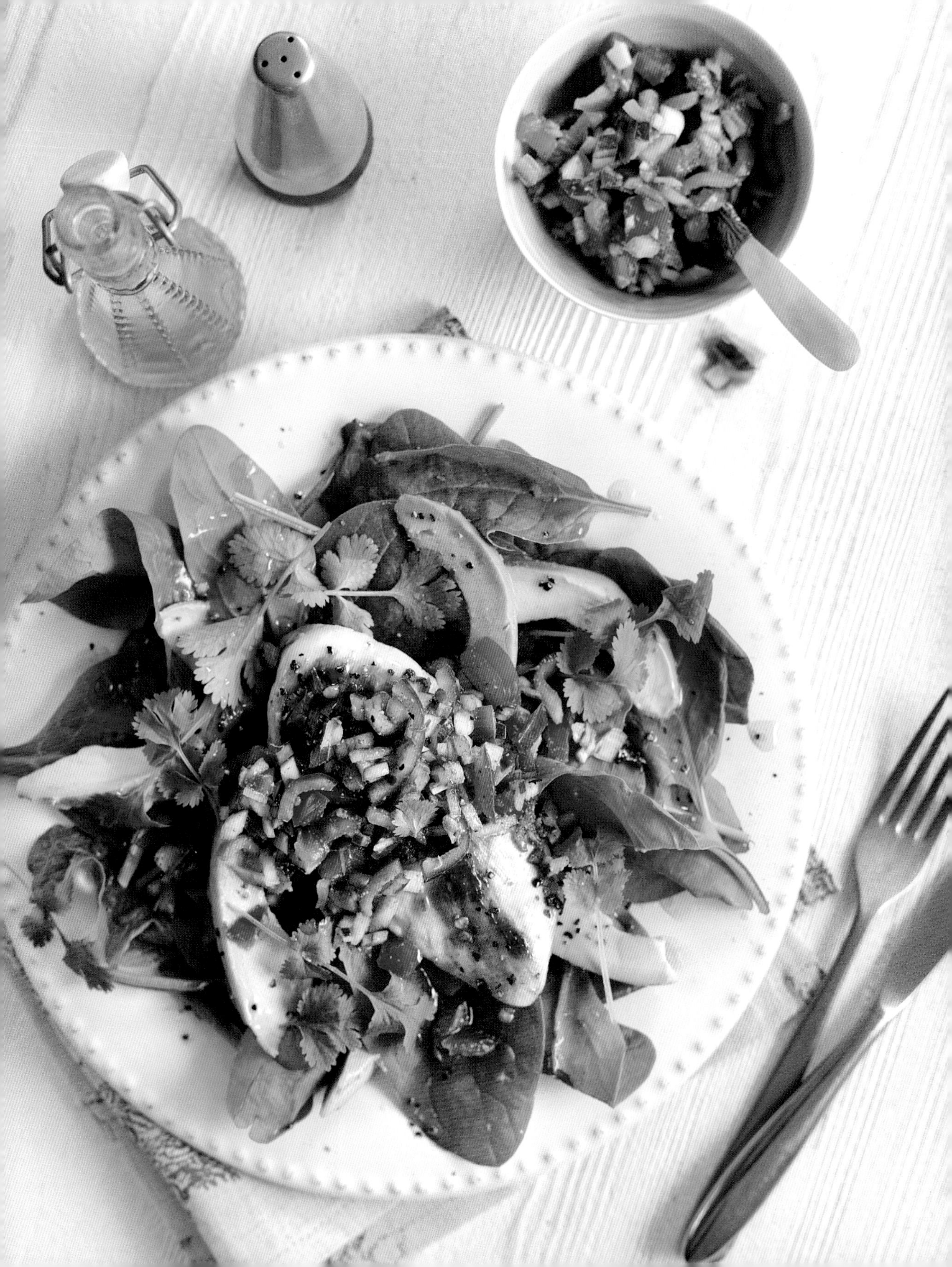

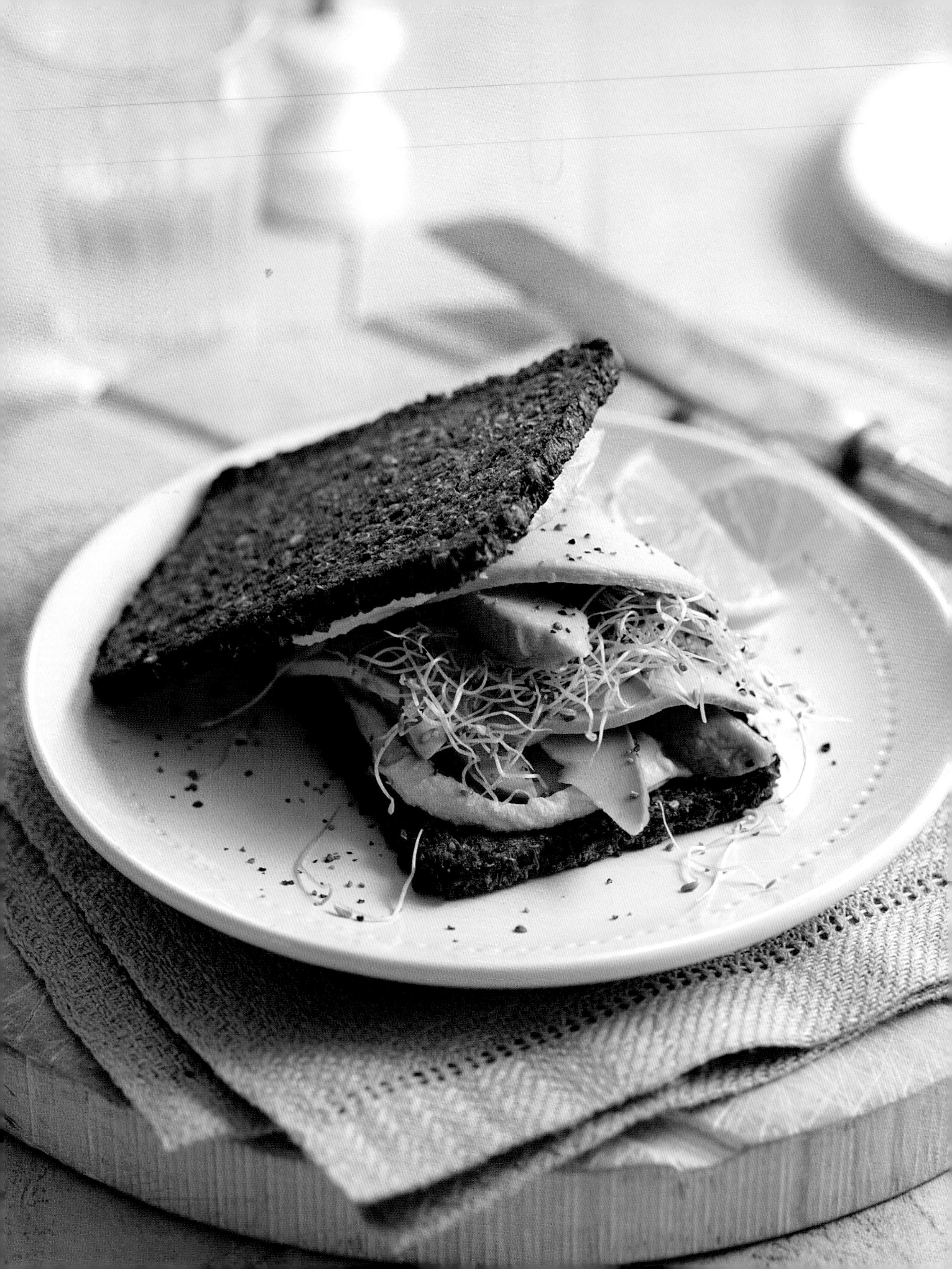

Green Clean & Lean Sandwich

Serves 1

Ingredients

2 slices rye bread
1 tablespoon hummus
juice of ½ lemon
2 slices cooked turkey
1 small ripe avocado, peeled and sliced
handful of alfalfa sprouts
freshly ground black pepper

Method

1 Toast the rye bread, spread the hummus over one side of each slice of toast, and sprinkle with the lemon juice.

2 Lay one slice of turkey, half the avocado, and half the alfafa sprouts over the hummus on each slice.

3 Season with freshly ground black pepper, and either sandwich 2 slices together or serve as an open sandwich.

Clean & Lean Guacamole

Serves 4

Ingredients

2 medium, ripe tomatoes
2 big ripe avocadoes
1 small red onion, chopped
½ small red chile, finely chopped (and seeded if you don't like it too hot)
1 tablespoon lemon or lime juice
½ teaspoon sea salt
freshly ground black pepper

Method

1 Remove the pulp and seeds from the tomatoes, cut into small dice, and set aside.

2 Scoop the avocado flesh into a bowl, add the onion, chile, juice, and salt, grind in some pepper, and mash everything together. Add the tomato and serve immediately.

Clean & Lean Hummus

Serves 4

Ingredients

1¼ cups chickpeas
3–5 tablespoons lemon juice, or to taste
1½ tablespoons tahini
2 garlic cloves, smashed
½ teaspoon sea salt
2 tablespoons olive oil, plus extra to drizzle later
½ tablespoon chopped parsley, to garnish (optional)

Method

1 Soak the chickpeas overnight in cold water. Drain, put in a pan, cover with fresh water, and boil under tender but not mushy. Drain, reserving the liquid, and allow to cool.

2 Put everything but the parsley in a blender, plus ½ cup of the reserved cooking liquid. Process until smooth.

3 Transfer to a bowl, drizzle in a little olive oil, and garnish with parsley.

*top tip

Avocados help to lower blood pressure because of all the monounsaturated fat and potassium they contain.

Clean & Lean Super Salad with Smoked Salmon

Serves 2

Ingredients

4 ounces baby spinach leaves
8–10 ripe cherry tomatoes
1 avocado, peeled and sliced
½ cucumber, diced
1 red pepper, seeded and diced
1 cup organic mung bean or mixed sprouts
2 tablespoons pumpkin seeds
2 tablespoons sunflower seeds
1 tablespoon pine nuts, toasted
extra virgin olive oil
2 ounces smoked salmon

Method

1 Divide the spinach, tomatoes and avocado between two plates. Sprinkle over the diced cucumber, red pepper, sprouts, seeds, and pine nuts, and drizzle with the olive oil.

2 Serve the smoked salmon alongside.

*top tip

You can vary the ingredients if you want, but remember that tomatoes are full of lycopene, which neutralizes the free radicals that damage the cells in the body.

*top tip

Nuts and seeds make a great snack. So do sliced white meats and vegetable sticks with Clean & Lean hummus or guacamole.

Cold Lamb Salad

Serves 4

Ingredients

4 slices cold, cooked lamb
4 large tomatoes, sliced
8 ounces mozzarella, sliced
olive oil, for drizzling
pinch of sea salt and freshly ground black pepper

Method

Simply arrange the ingredients on a plate, season with a twist of pepper, and drizzle olive oil over the salad.

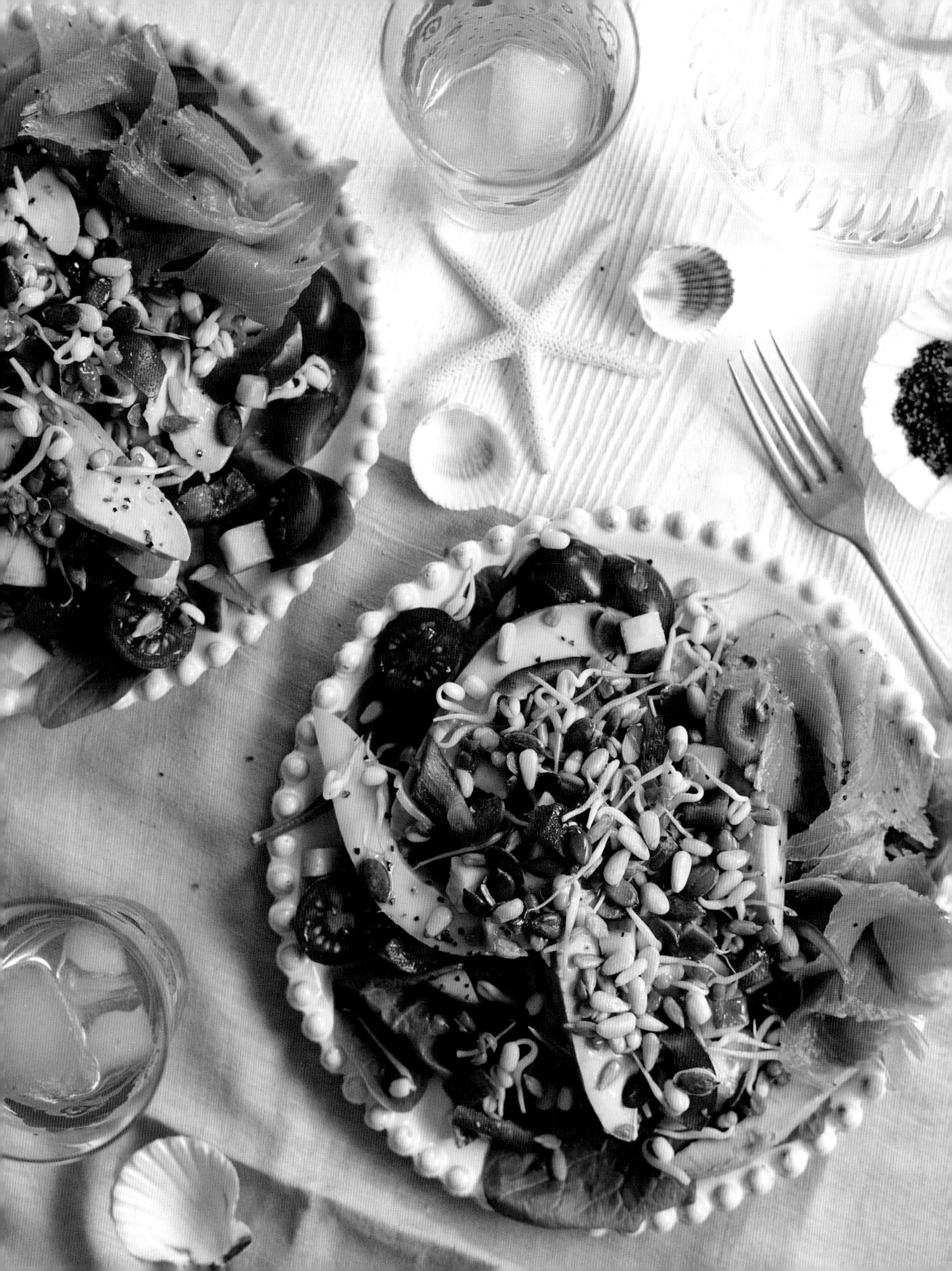

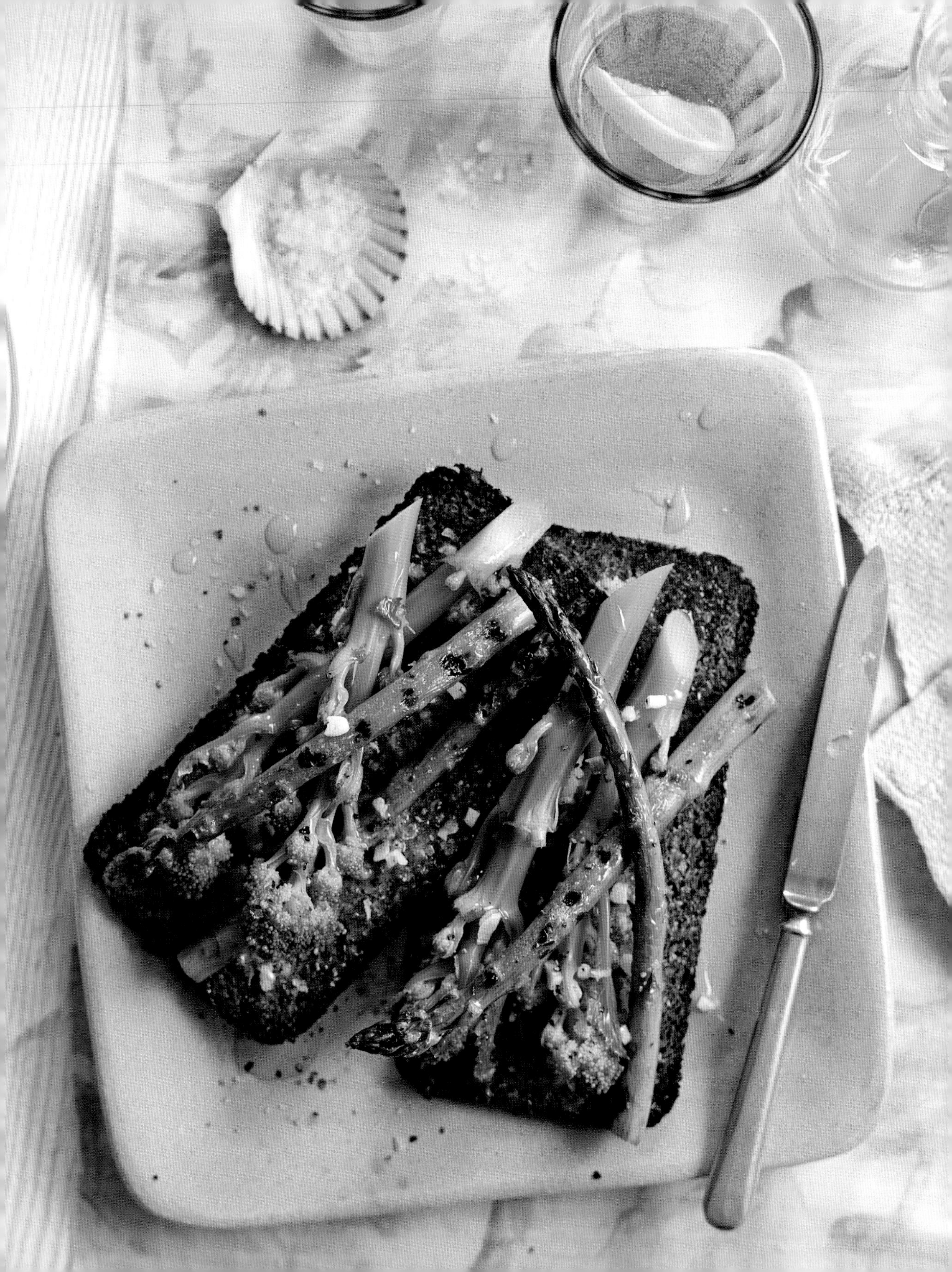

*top tip

Add some crumbled goat cheese for extra protein!

Rye Bruschetta with Broccoli and Asparagus

Serves 2

Ingredients

8 small heads broccolini, halved lengthwise
8 asparagus spears
4 slices rye bread
2 garlic cloves, smashed
olive oil
salt and freshly ground black pepper
1 garlic clove, roughly chopped

Method

1 Steam the broccolini until just tender. Grill the asparagus. Keep warm.

2 Toast the rye bread slices and rub them with the smashed garlic cloves. Drizzle with a little olive oil, and arrange the broccolini and asparagus on top. Season with salt and pepper and the chopped garlic clove.

Cannellini Bean and Rosemary Dip

Serves 4

Ingredients

1 cup cannellini beans
juice of 1 lemon
1 garlic clove, crushed
½ cup organic Greek yogurt
handful of rosemary leaves
handful of chia seeds
sea salt and freshly ground black pepper

Method

1 Soak the beans overnight in cold water. Drain, put in a pan, cover with fresh water, and boil until tender but not mushy. Drain, and allow to cool.

2 Put the beans in a food processor or blender with the lemon juice, garlic, yogurt, and rosemary leaves, and process until smooth. Stir in the chia seeds and season with salt and freshly ground black pepper.

3 Serve with sticks of carrot and celery for dipping.

*top tip

For vegetarians, protein is very important for developing lean muscle that helps you burn fat constantly. I recommend a good-quality protein powder such as Protein Excellence, which can be mixed with water or milk. Other good foods are a combination of rice or hemp protein, tempeh, fermented tofu, lentils and beans, eggs, and dairy.

Quinoa and Roasted Pepper Salad with Seeds

Serves 2

Ingredients

2 red peppers, seeded and cut into quarters
1 garlic clove, chopped
1 tablespoon freshly chopped parsley
1½ tablespoons extra virgin olive oil
salt and freshly ground black pepper
½ cup quinoa, rinsed and drained
2 teaspoons balsamic vinegar
2 tomatoes, chopped
1 red onion, finely chopped
2 tablespoons sunflower seeds
2 tablespoons chia seeds

Method

1 Preheat the oven to 425°F. Place the peppers on a baking sheet, cut side up. Scatter with the chopped garlic and parsley, and drizzle with half the olive oil. Season with sea salt and freshly ground black pepper. Place the baking sheet in the oven and roast for 20 minutes.

2 Meanwhile, cook the quinoa according to the packeage instructions, then drain well and place in a bowl. Whisk together the remaining olive oil and the balsamic vinegar, then stir into the quinoa and fluff with a fork. Finally, mix in the tomatoes and red onion and serve with the roasted pepper. Scatter the seeds over the top.

Salad of Wild Rice, Fish, Spiced Pecans, and Avocado

Serves 4

Ingredients

½ cup wild rice
1 small cinnamon stick
1 red chile, split lengthwise
½ red onion, finely chopped
2 tablespoons olive oil
1½ tablespoons good-quality red wine vinegar
¼ teaspoon sweet smoked paprika
½ cup pecans
½ teaspoon cumin seeds
4 mackerel or salmon fillets
½ tablespoon freshly chopped cilantro
1 ripe avocado, cut into pieces
a small bunch of watercress, washed

Method

1 Preheat the oven to 300°F.

2 Simmer the wild rice, cinnamon, and chile in plenty of water until tender but still al dente, and drain (check your package of wild rice for timings, and taste for tenderness). Leave to cool.

3 Cook the red onion in a pan in 1 tablespoon of the oil until soft. Add the vinegar and paprika, and continue to cook until the vinegar has evaporated. Remove from the heat and allow to cool.

4 Toss the pecans with the cumin seeds, salt, and 1 tablespoon water. Bake for 10 minutes or until golden (keep checking to make sure they don't burn).

5 Meanwhile, score the skin of the mackerel fillets and season both sides with salt and pepper. Heat a heavy-bottomed frying pan and drizzle the skin of the fish with the remaining olive oil. Sear skin-side down first for 2–3 minutes, then flip and repeat on the flesh side.

6 Mix the rice, onion, cilantro, avocado, and watercress together, and arrange on 4 plates. Place a mackerel fillet on top, and sprinkle with the pecans to serve.

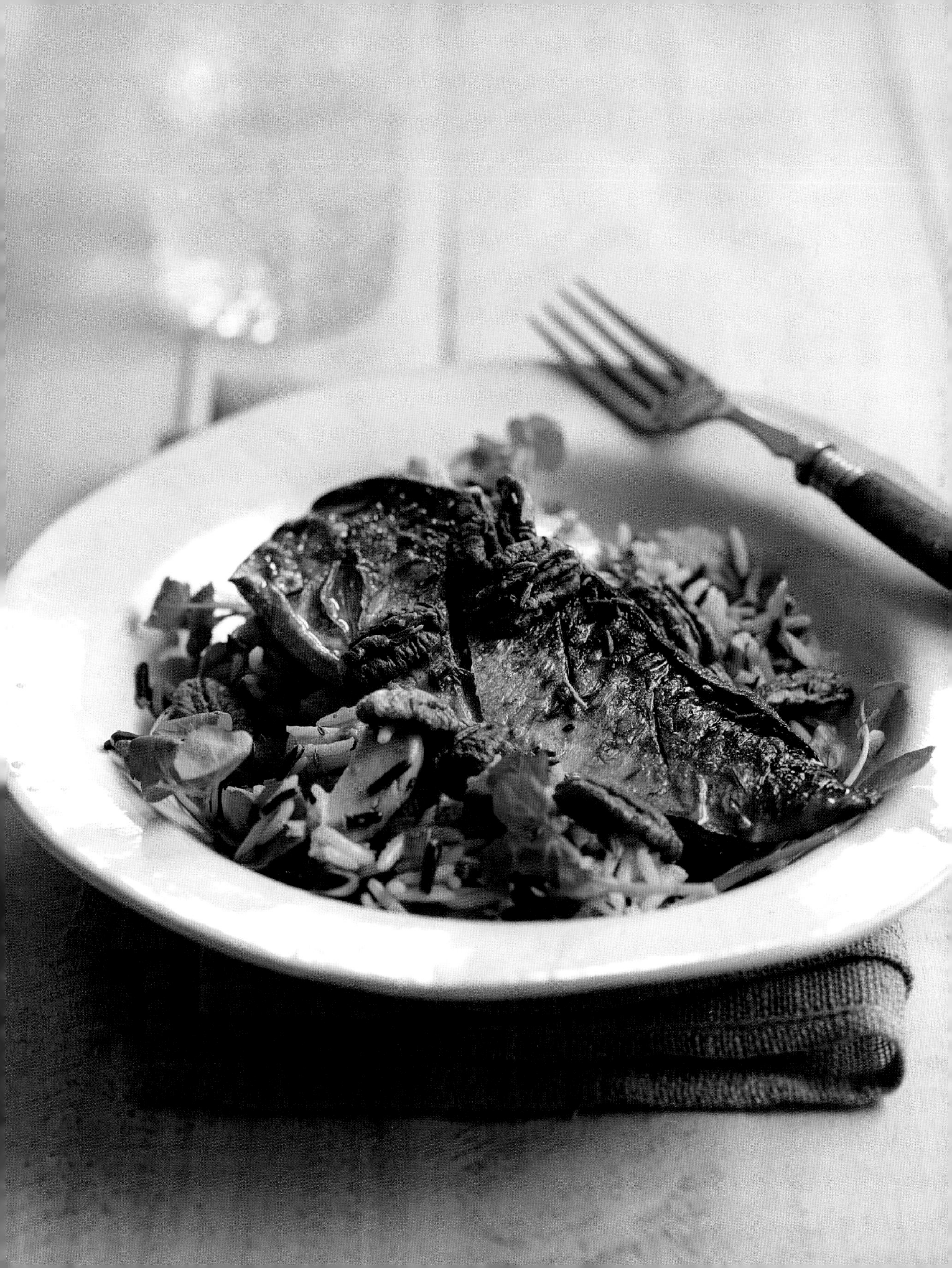

Spicy Beet and Lamb Salad

Serves 4

Ingredients

You will need 4 wooden skewers, soaked in water for 30 minutes
1⅔ lbs trimmed beets
1 lb lean lamb, diced into large chunks
2 zucchini, cut into thick rounds
2 red onions, cut into quarters
4 tablespoons olive oil
1 garlic clove, crushed
sea salt and freshly ground black pepper
juice of ½ lemon
½ teaspoon ground cumin
½ teaspoon ground cinnamon
½ teaspoon ground paprika
1 tablespoon orange flower water
2 tablespoons freshly chopped parsley
4 large handfuls of arugula

Method

1 Cook the beets in a steamer for 20–30 minutes until tender. Set aside to cool.

2 Meanwhile, toss the lamb pieces, zucchini, and red onions in 2 tablespoons of the olive oil, along with the garlic and some salt and pepper. Thread onto the prepared skewers, alternating the lamb, zucchini, and red onions.

3 When the beets have cooled, peel and slice them, reserving the liquid that accumulates on the plate. Toss them in the juice of the lemon and coat with the cumin, cinnamon, paprika, orange flower water, and remaining olive oil, together with the reserved beet liquid.

4 Season with salt and black pepper, cover, and chill.

5 Preheat the broiler to high. Cook the lamb skewers under the broiler for 7–10 minutes, before turning and repeating. Check to make sure the lamb is cooked to your liking.

6 To serve, toss the beets with the parsley and arrange with the arugula on plates. Serve the lamb skewers alongside.

Red and Yellow Pepper Spelt Salad

Serves 2

Ingredients

½ cup pearled spelt
½ red pepper, chopped into large chunks
½ yellow pepper, chopped into large chunks
½ head of broccoli, broken into florets
1½ tablespoons olive oil
1 teaspoon white wine vinegar
1 garlic clove, crushed
sea salt and freshly ground black pepper
freshly chopped basil leaves, to garnish

Method

1 Boil the spelt for 15–20 minutes, or according to package instructions, until just tender. Drain well and leave to cool.

2 Meanwhile, preheat the broiler. Place the pepper chunks on a sheet of foil on a broiler pan and broil for about 5–10 minutes until charred and blistered, then set aside.

3 Steam the broccoli for 3–4 minutes until just cooked, and set aside.

4 Whisk together the olive oil, white wine vinegar, garlic, salt and freshly ground black pepper, and pour over the spelt. Stir well, then allow to cool. Once cool, add the peppers and some freshly chopped basil leaves and stir. Check the seasoning and serve at room temperature with a grilled chicken breast or piece of fish.

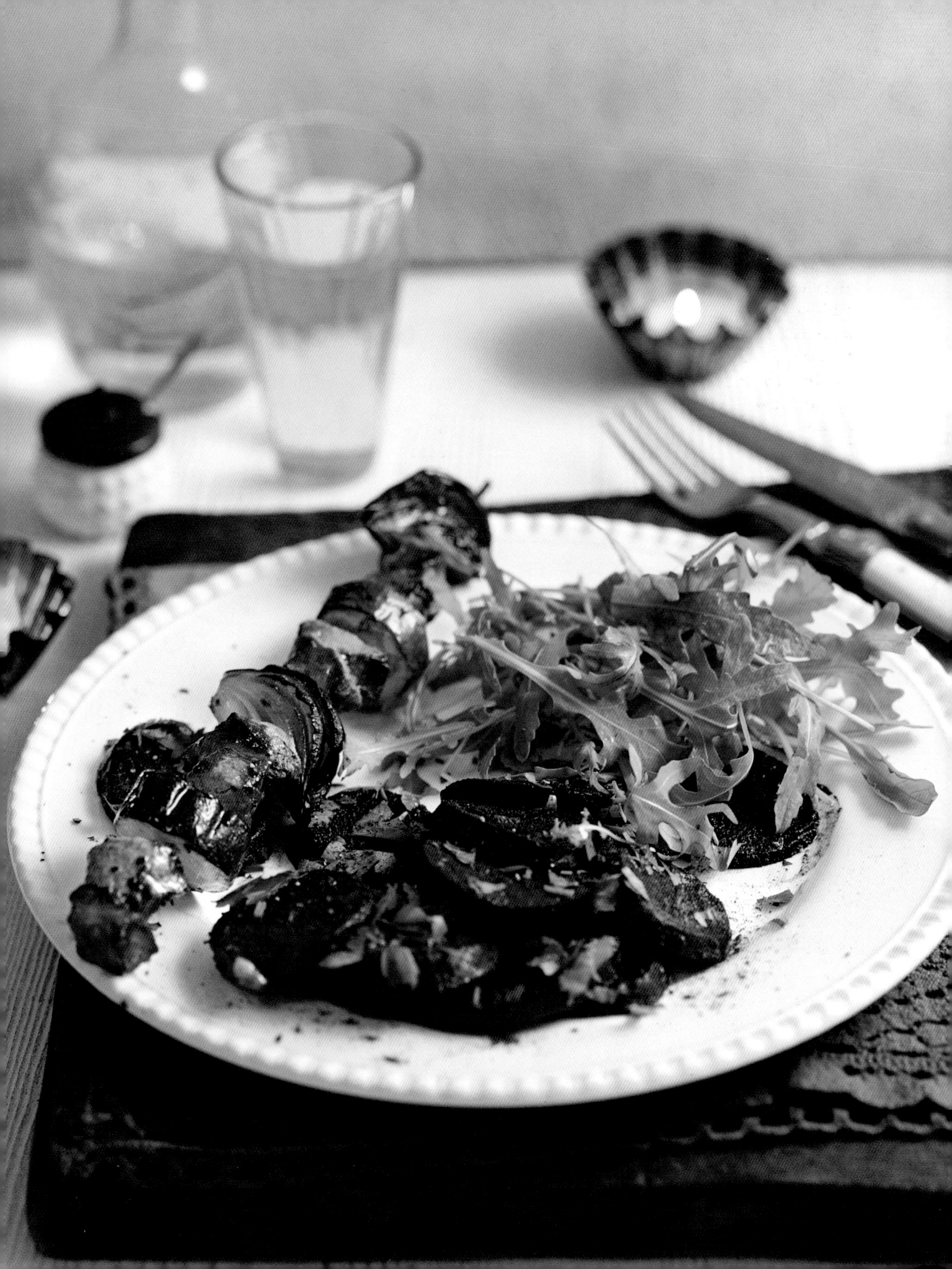

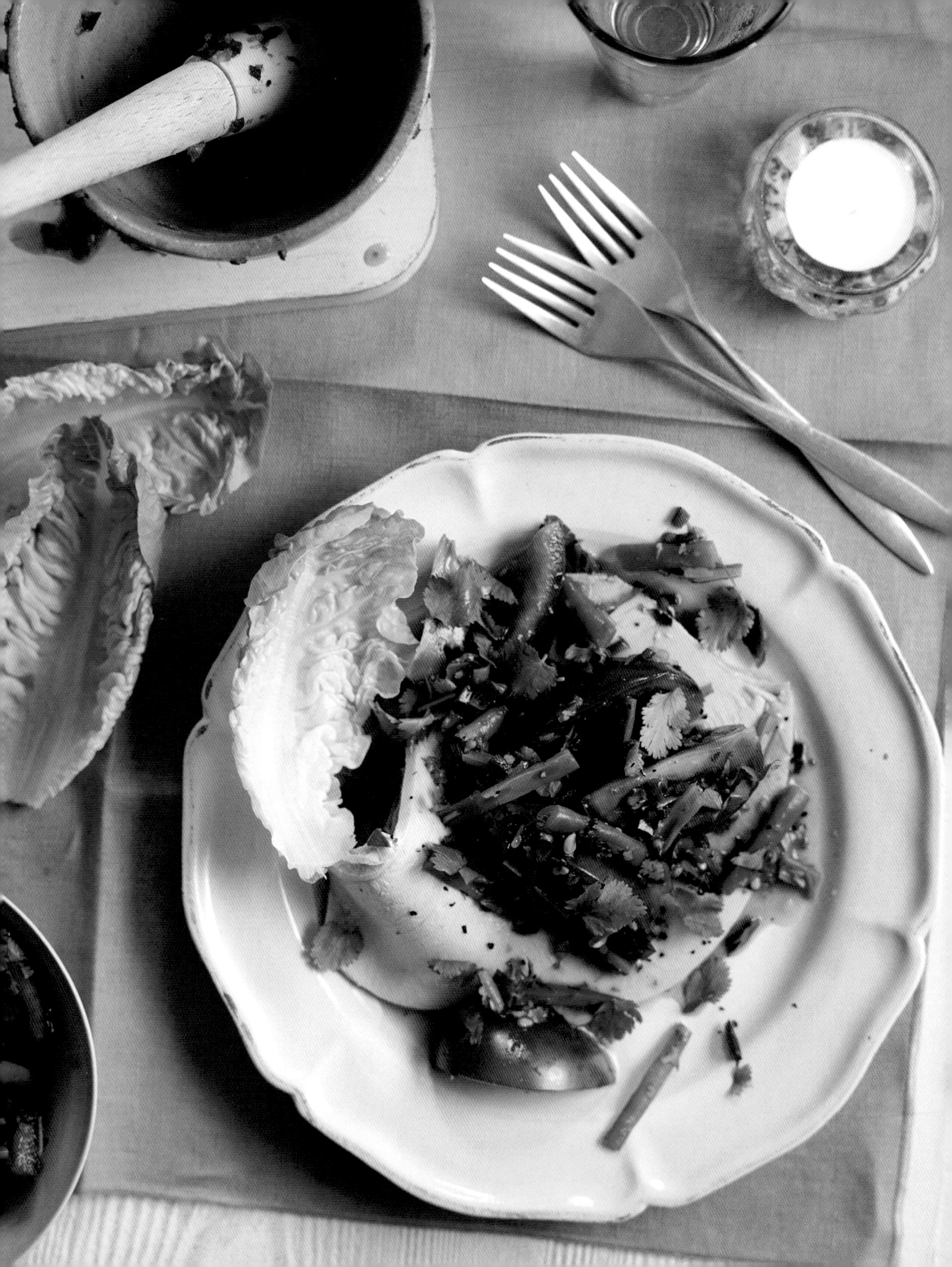

*top tip

Just one ounce of spinach gives you 40 percent of your daily magnesium requirement (insufficient magnesium leads to headaches and fatigue).

Green Bean and Tomato Salad with Turkey

Serves 2

Ingredients

20 green beans, chopped into 2-inch lengths
2 garlic cloves, peeled
3–4 small fresh red or green chiles, chopped
4 ripe tomatoes, cut into wedges
2 tablespoons lime juice
8 ounces cooked turkey, sliced
handful of cilantro leaves
Boston lettuce leaves, to serve

Method

1 Steam or boil the beans until tender, then drain.

2 Pound the garlic in a large mortar, then add the chiles and pound again. Add the beans, breaking them up slightly, then pour into a bowl. Add the tomato and lightly mash.

3 Drizzle in the lime juice, and transfer to a serving dish. Scatter with the sliced turkey and cilantro leaves. Serve with Boston lettuce leaves, which can be used as a scoop for the mixture.

Lima Bean, Spinach, and Turkey Salad

Serves 4

Ingredients

1 cup lima beans or edamame, fresh or frozen
1 tablespoon olive oil
1 teaspoon white wine vinegar
salt and freshly ground black pepper
½ cup feta, crumbled
1 cup baby spinach
8 ounces cooked turkey, sliced
fresh mint leaves, to garnish

Method

1 Bring a large pan of water to a boil, put in the lima beans, and blanch them for 2–3 minutes, then drain and refresh in iced water. Peel off the outer skins of the beans if necessary.

2 Whisk together the olive oil and white wine vinegar. Season the beans with salt and freshly ground black pepper, and stir in half of the vinaigrette.

3 Arrange the beans on a plate along with the feta, spinach, and turkey, and drizzle with the remaining vinaigrette. Garnish with the fresh mint leaves.

Grilled Rib-Eye Steak with Sweet Potato Mash and Chile Broccoli

Serves 4

Ingredients

2 small sweet potatoes, peeled and roughly chopped
2 tablespoons organic Greek yogurt
3 tablespoons pomegranate seeds
sea salt and freshly ground black pepper
4 x 8 ounce grass-fed rib-eye steaks
2 tablespoons sesame oil, plus extra for drizzling
1 large broccoli, broken into florets
1 small red chile, finely sliced

Method

1 Place the sweet potatoes in a medium saucepan and just cover with water. Bring to boil and cook, uncovered, for about 8 minutes or until very soft. Drain and transfer to a large bowl and mash with the yogurt, then stir in the pomegranate seeds and season to taste.

2 Meanwhile, heat a grill pan until very hot. Rub the steaks with 2 tablespoons of the sesame oil and season. Cook for about 3 minutes on each side for medium-rare. Leave to rest for 5–10 minutes.

3 Steam the broccoli, then transfer to a bowl. Drizzle with the remaining sesame oil, and sprinkle with the sliced chile.

4 Serve the steak with the mashed sweet potato and broccoli on the side.

Spelt Risotto with Butternut Squash, Arugula, Walnuts, and Goat Cheese

Serves 4

Ingredients

1 squash (such as butternut or acorn), weighing about 1½ lbs, peeled, seeded and cut into chunks
8 sage leaves, chopped, plus extra to garnish
2 garlic cloves, smashed
2 tablespoons olive oil
1 red onion, chopped
1 cup pearled spelt
3 cups hot vegetable stock
2 handfuls of arugula
½ cup walnuts, toasted and roughly chopped
2 ounces hard goat cheese
salt and freshly ground black pepper

Method

1 Preheat the oven to 375°F.

2 Put the butternut squash into a roasting pan, add the chopped sage and garlic, season, and drizzle with half the olive oil. Roast for about 25 minutes until tender and starting to brown at the edges.

3 Meanwhile, start making the risotto. Heat the remaining oil in a large sauté pan over a medium heat. Add the onion and cook until soft. Add the spelt and stir into the onions. Continue to cook for 1 minute until the spelt starts to smell slightly nutty.

4 Pour ⅔ cup of the stock into the pan, stirring all the time. Allow most of it to evaporate, and then add the rest of the stock a ladleful at a time, stirring frequently until all the liquid has been absorbed and the spelt is tender but still has some "bite."

5 Add the roasted butternut squash, arugula, and walnuts to the pan. Stir to combine, and season to taste with salt and freshly ground black pepper. Using a vegetable peeler, shave the goat cheese over the risotto, garnish with sage, and serve immediately.

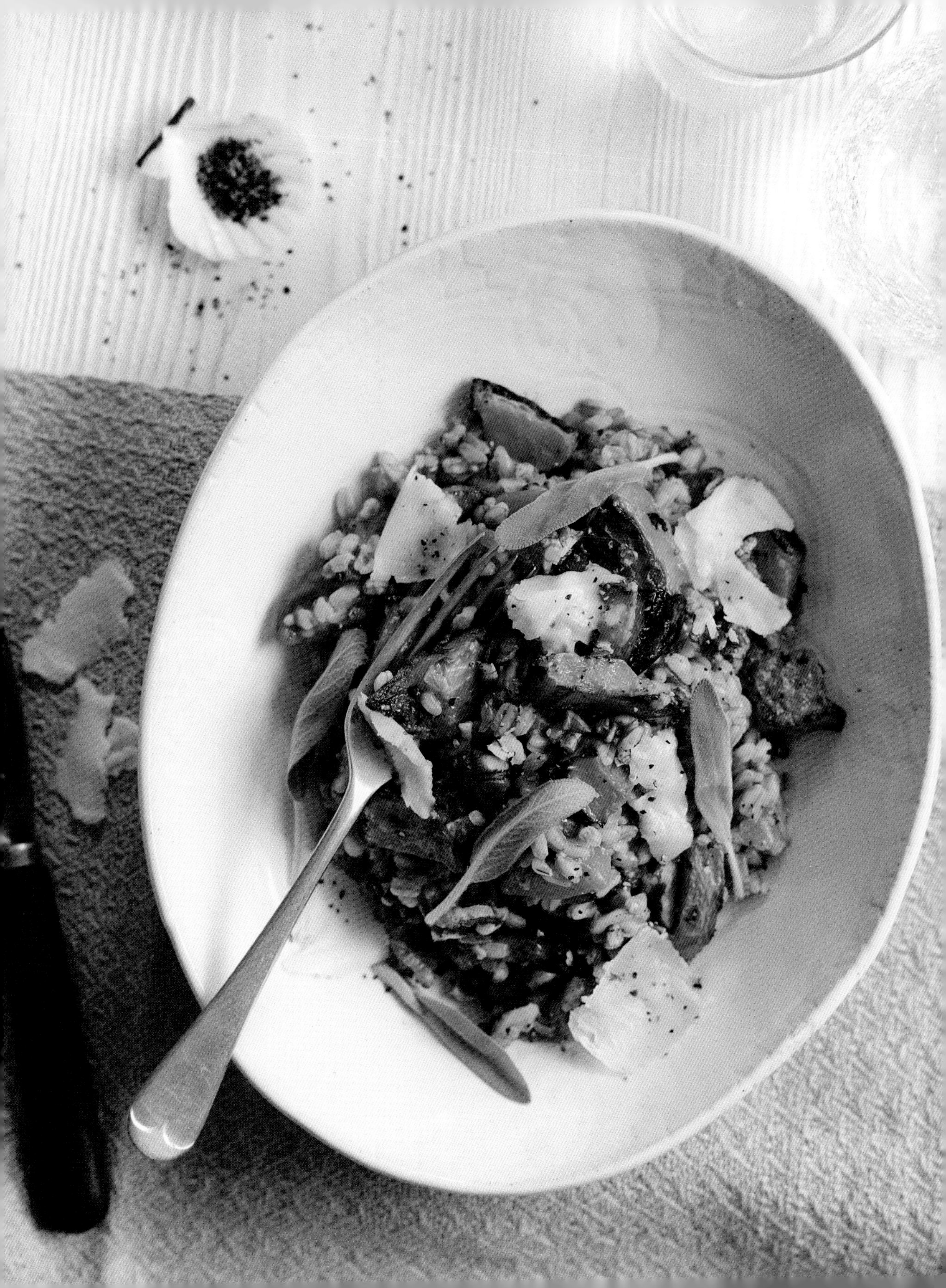

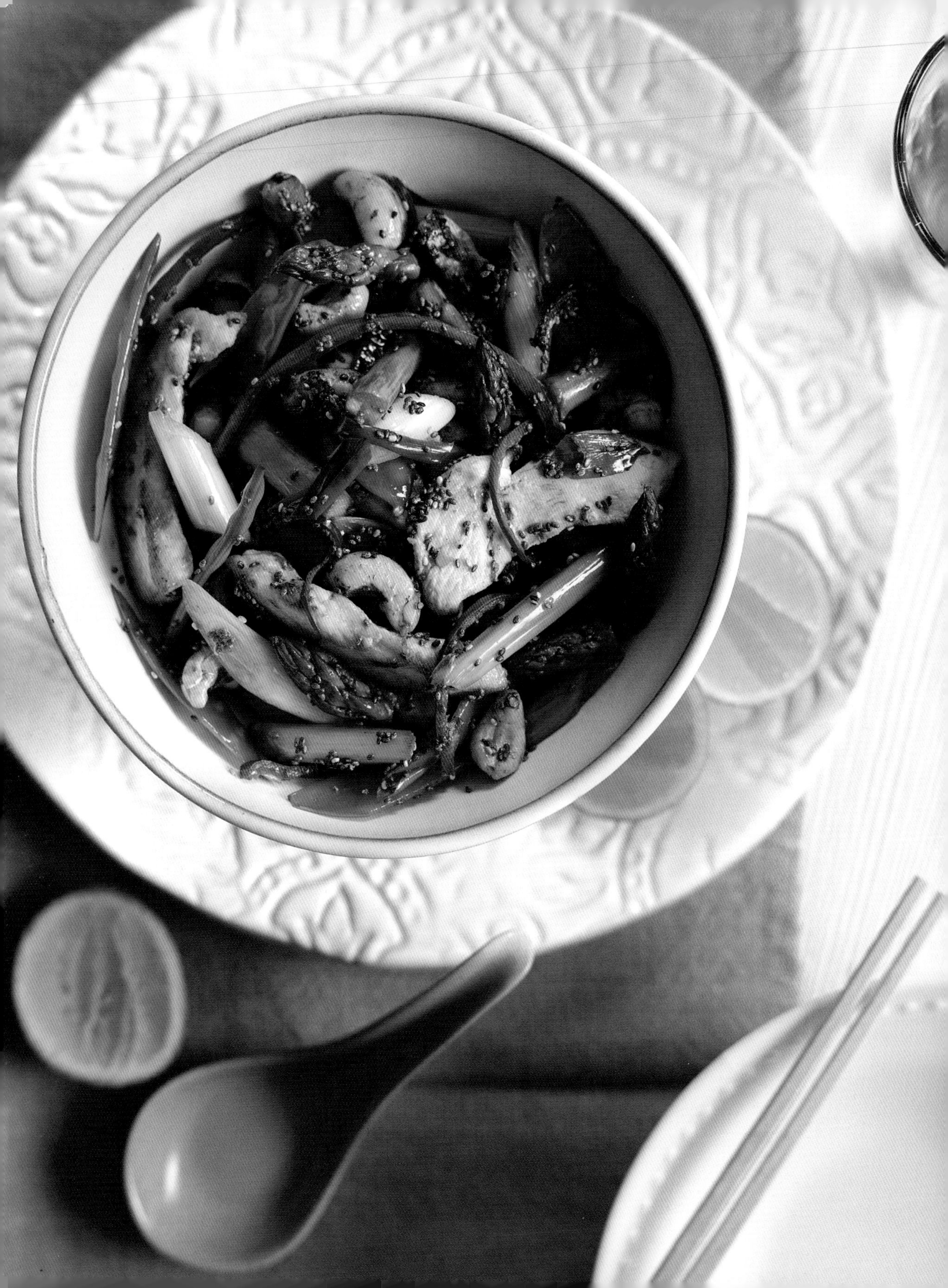

Chicken, Asparagus, and Cashew Stir-fry

Serves 4

Ingredients

2 skinless organic chicken breast fillets, cut into ½-inch thick strips
3 tablespoons vegetable oil
2 cloves garlic, smashed
½ cup unsalted cashews
2 long red chiles, thinly sliced
6 scallions, sliced
8 ounces asparagus, cut into bite-size pieces
8 ounces snow peas or sugar snaps, topped, tailed, and sliced lengthwise
⅓ cup chicken stock
2 tablespoons chia seeds
juice of 1 lime

Method

1 Heat a wok over high heat. Add half the oil and, when hot, add the chicken, garlic, and cashews, and stir-fry for 3–4 minutes or until the chicken is almost cooked through. Remove from the wok and set aside.

2 Pour in the remaining oil. Add the chiles, scallions, snow peas or sugar snap peas, and broccoli, and stir-fry for 2 minutes. Add the stock and stir-fry for 2 minutes more.

3 Return the chicken, garlic and cashews to the wok, and stir-fry until heated through. Stir in the chia seeds. Add the lime juice and serve immediately.

*top tip

This super bolognese is cheap, easy, and bursting with nutrition. You can also use any vegetables you have in your fridge.

Super Bolognese Sauce

Serves 4

Ingredients

1 red onion
1 red pepper
1 zucchini
⅓ cup peas (fresh or frozen)
1½ cups broccoli florets
2 celery ribs
1 eggplant
1 tablespoon olive oil
1 lb lean organic ground beef
1⅔ cups organic tomato sauce
2 cloves garlic, smashed
1 tablespoon chopped fresh rosemary
sea salt
freshly ground black pepper
1 tablespoon chopped parsley

Method

1 Chop all the vegetables into equal-sized chunks.

2 Heat the olive oil in a large lidded pan, and cook the ground beef until browned. Add the vegetables, tomato sauce, garlic, and rosemary, season with salt and pepper, and simmer for 30–45 minutes, or until the vegetables are tender.

3 Serve sprinkled with the chopped parsley. If you want, you can accompany it with a little brown rice or spelt pasta (but I prefer it without).

*top tip

Choose your seafood wisely Overfishing and its impact on our oceans is a serious concern. Make sustainable seafood choices by doing your research. A good resource is fishtofork.com Also, ask your fishmongers where they source their produce from.

Lemon and Chile Broccoli

Serves 2 as a side

Ingredients

1 teaspoon olive oil
1 garlic clove, sliced
3 cups blanched broccoli
zest and juice of ½ lemon
1 red chile, finely sliced
handful of sunflower seeds
handful of pumpkin seeds
1 tablespoon chia seeds
sea salt and freshly ground black pepper

Method

Heat the olive oil in a large pan, and cook the garlic until softened. Add the broccoli, lemon zest, and juice, and heat through. Stir in the chile and seeds, and season to taste.

Salmon en Papillote with Ginger and Lime

Serves 4

Ingredients

2-inch piece ginger, peeled and thinly sliced
2 cloves garlic
4 scallions, finely sliced
1 red chile, finely sliced
4 salmon fillets
juice of 1 lime
1 lime, thinly sliced
4 sheets of parchment paper, each large enough to fold over the salmon and form a parcel

Method

1 Preheat the oven to 400°F.

2 Mix the ginger, garlic, scallions, and chile together in a bowl.

3 Place each piece of salmon in the center of a sheet of parchment paper, and top with a quarter of the ginger mixture. Sprinkle each fillet with lime juice and then top with a few slices of lime.

4 Fold the parchment paper over each fillet, and tuck the edges in to form a parcel.

5 Place the parcels on a baking sheet and bake for around 12 minutes.

*top tip

Serve with a pile of fresh, green, stir-fried vegetables—packed with vitamins that help to replenish a stressed body.

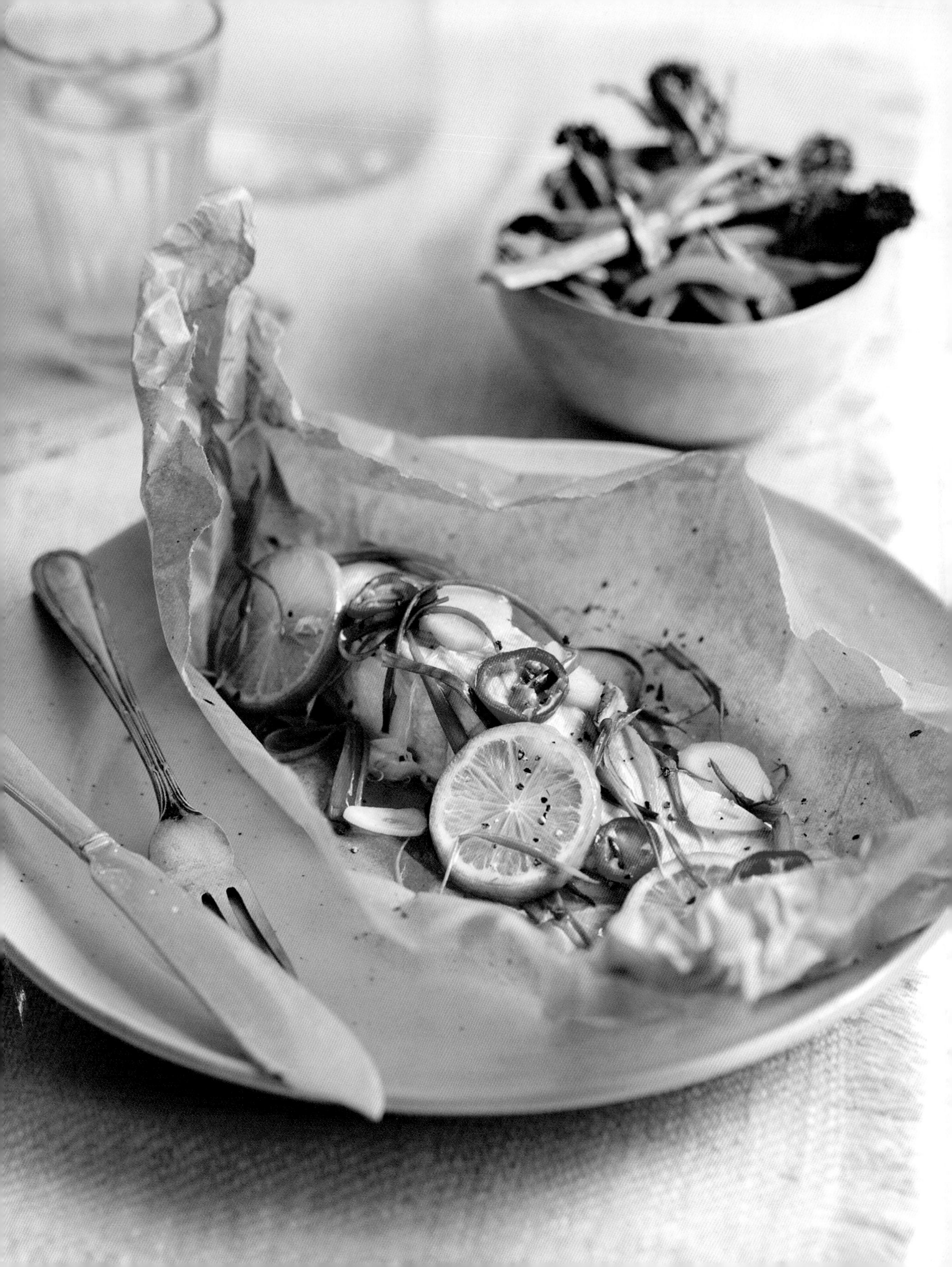

DESSERTS

Roasted Peaches with Honey and Yogurt

Serves 4

Ingredients

4 ripe peaches, halved and pitted
juice of 2 oranges
1 tablespoon Manuka honey
½ cup Greek yogurt
1 teaspoon vanilla extract
⅓ cup chopped pistachios, to garnish

Method

1 Preheat the oven to 400°F.

2 Set the peach halves cut side up in a roasting pan. Pour the orange juice around them, and then drizzle the cut surfaces with the honey. Roast for 10–15 minutes.

3 Meanwhile, combine the yogurt with the vanilla. Place the peach halves in individual bowls, spoon on some yogurt, and scatter with the pistachios.

*top tip

Yogurt neutralizes the acidity caused by stress. Don't go for the low-fat, flavored stuff—choose a plain, organic one.

Melon with Cinnamon and Nutty Yogurt

Serves 4

Ingredients

1 honeydew melon, cut into quarters with the seeds removed
1 teaspoon ground cinnamon
1 cup organic Greek yogurt

For the nuts

1 tablespoon organic butter
1 tablespoon Manuka honey
½ cup walnuts
½ teaspoon ground cinnamon

Method

1 First make the nutty yogurt: melt the butter in a saucepan over low heat, and stir in the honey until combined. Add the walnuts and cinnamon, and stir until the walnuts are coated. Spread the walnuts out on a baking sheet lined with parchment paper, and let cool.

2 Score the melon so that it is easy to break into bite-size chunks, and sprinkle with the cinnamon.

3 Stir the candied walnuts into the yogurt and serve alongside the melon.

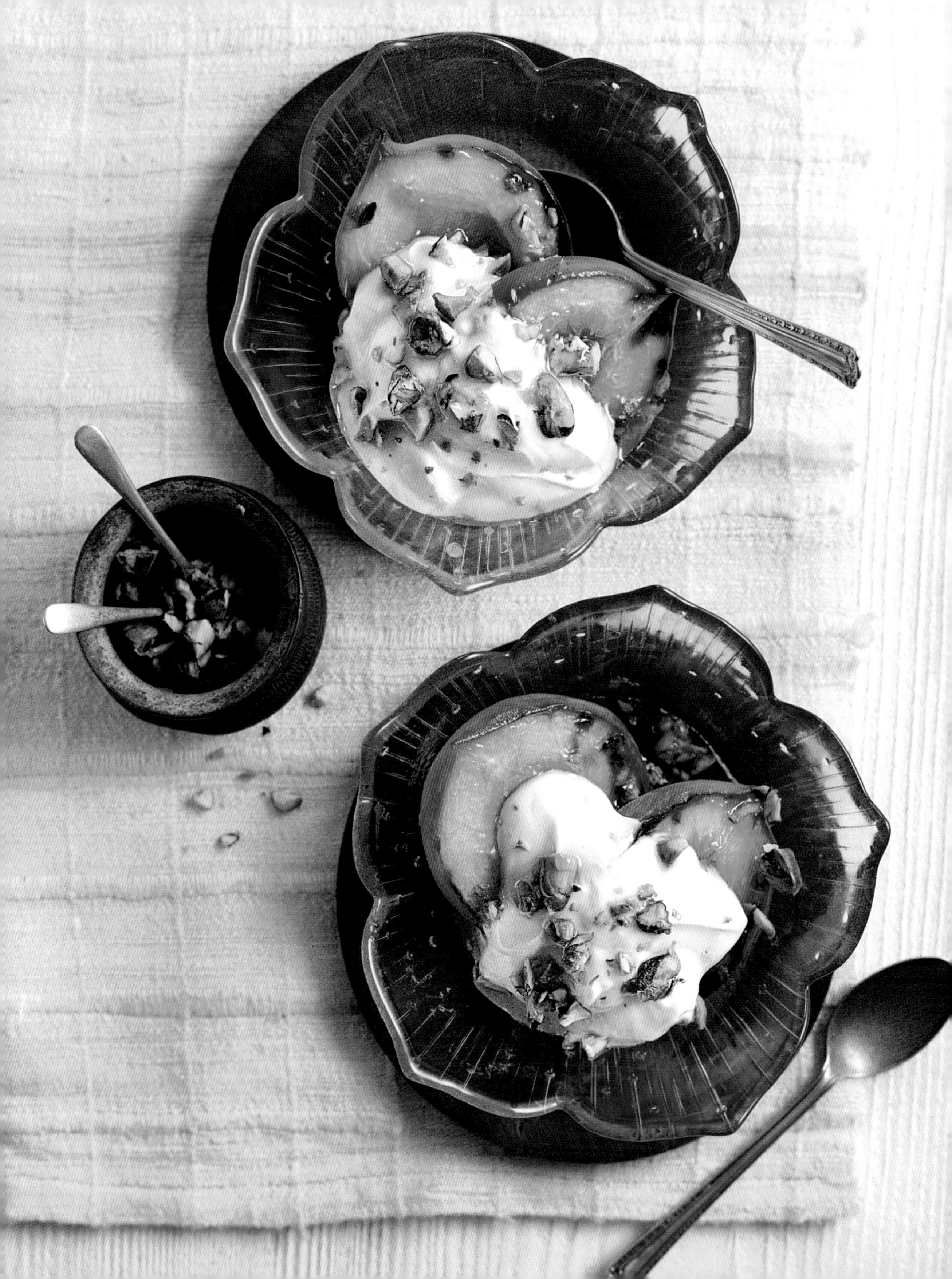

Peach, Melon, and Kiwi Salad

Serves 4

Ingredients

2 ripe peaches, sliced
2 kiwi fruit, peeled and sliced
1 small cantaloupe or honeydew melon
juice of 1 lemon
juice of 1 orange
2 tablespoons Manuka honey
large handful of fresh mint, torn
4 tablespoons organic Greek yogurt, to serve

Method

1 Place the peaches and kiwi fruit in a bowl. Halve the melon and scoop out the seeds. Cut the flesh into bite-size pieces and add to the bowl.

2 Whisk together the lemon and orange juice. Pour over the fruit and gently toss. Drizzle with the Manuka honey and scatter the torn mint leaves over the top. Serve with a dollop of Greek yogurt.

*top tip

Kiwis contain more vitamin C than an orange and as much potassium as a banana.

Watermelon, Feta, Mint, and Honey

Serves 4

Ingredients

4 large slices watermelon
8 ounces feta cheese, cut into cubes
handful of fresh mint
Manuka honey, to serve

Method

1 Arrange the slices of watermelon and feta on a serving dish or on 4 separate plates.

2 Scatter with the mint leaves, and drizzle with a little honey. Serve immediately.

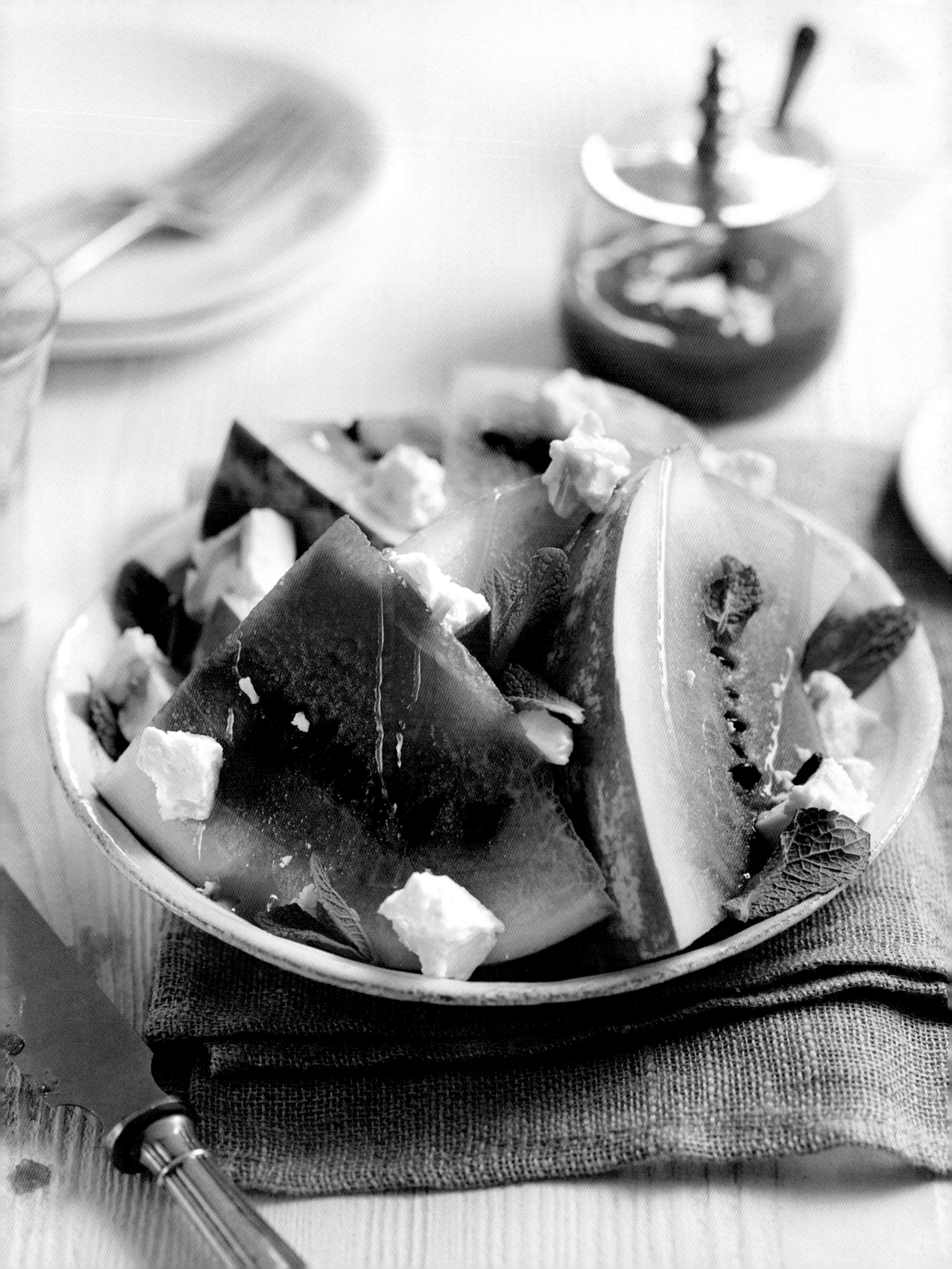

Fruit & Seed Crumble

Serves 6-8

Ingredients

For the topping

1¼ cups oats
¾ cup mixed seeds (pumpkin, sunflower)
1 cup pecans
¼ cup Brazil nuts
½ cup almonds
1 tablespoon chia seeds
½ teaspoon ground fennel seeds
grated zest and juice of 1 orange
½ teaspoon cinnamon
3 tablespoons agave syrup

For the fruit

4 large organic apples
1 pear
1 cup blackberries
1 tablespoon coconut oil
2 tablespoons water
1 teaspoon pure vanilla extract
½ teaspoon cinnamon
2 teaspoons Manuka honey

Method

1 Preheat the oven to 350°F.

2 Make the topping by combining all the ingredients in a bowl.

3 To make the filling, chop the fruit into small chunks. Heat the oil, water, and fruit in a pan until the fruit becomes soft, then add the vanilla, cinnamon, and honey, and heat until the mixture has thickened a little.

4 Transfer to an baking dish, cover with the topping mixture, and bake in the preheated oven for around 30 minutes.

5 Serve with plain organic yogurt.

Poached Pears Dipped in Chocolate

Serves 4

Ingredients

4 ripe pears, peeled, cored ,and halved
4 ounces dark chocolate
½ cup almonds, crushed

Method

1 Place the pears in a pan, cover with water, and poach very gently for 8–10 minutes until tender, then drain.

2 Melt the chocolate in a bowl over a pan of simmering water.

3 Place the crushed almonds in a bowl, and have 4 serving bowls ready.

4 Dip each pear in the chocolate until lightly coated, then in the almonds so that the almonds stick to the chocolate. Serve immediately.

*top tip

Chocolate can act as a mood elevator, and it contains magnesium, which soothes fragile nerves. However, to cut down on sugar, keep it as a treat, and buy the high-quality, organic kind.

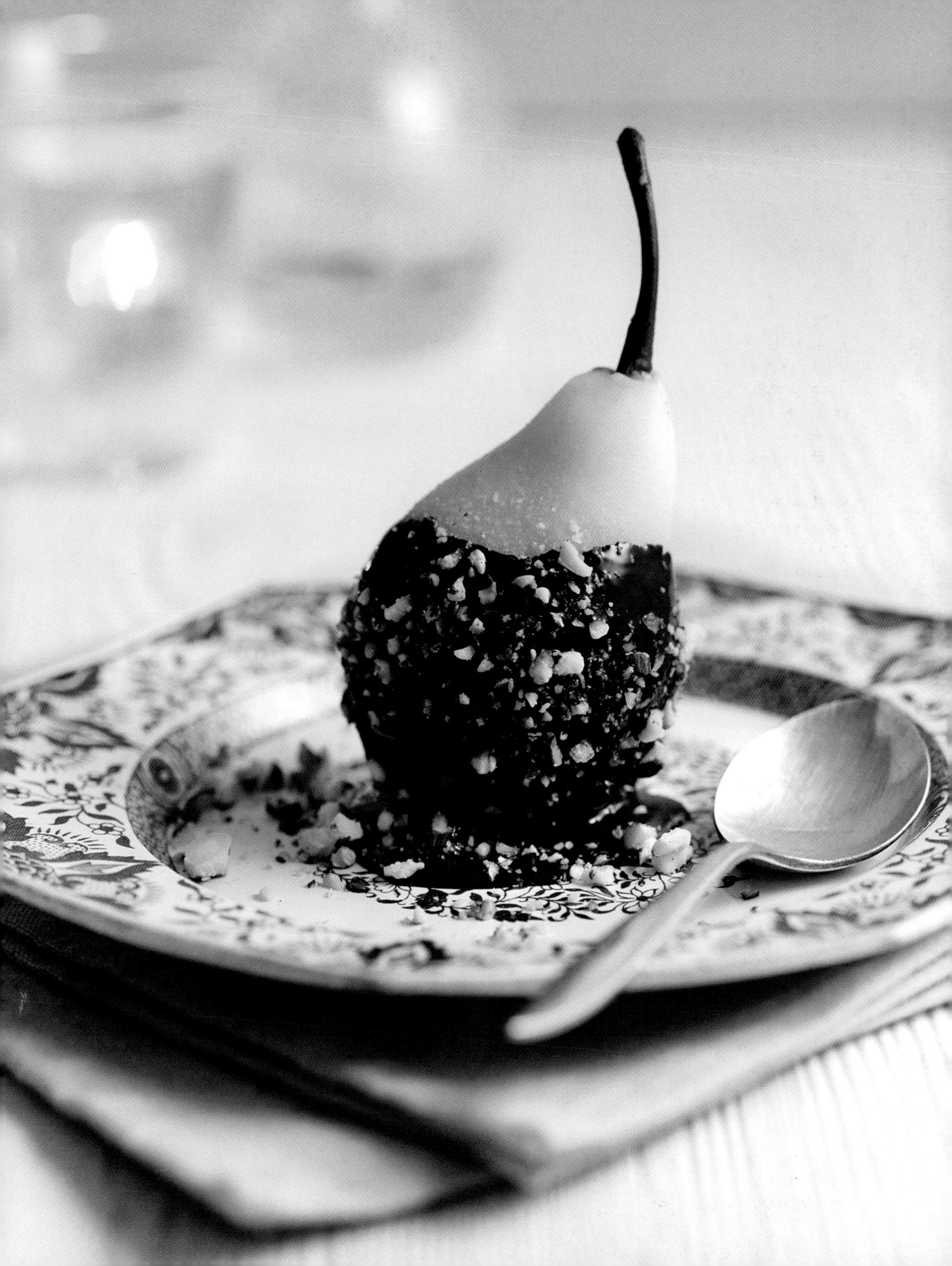

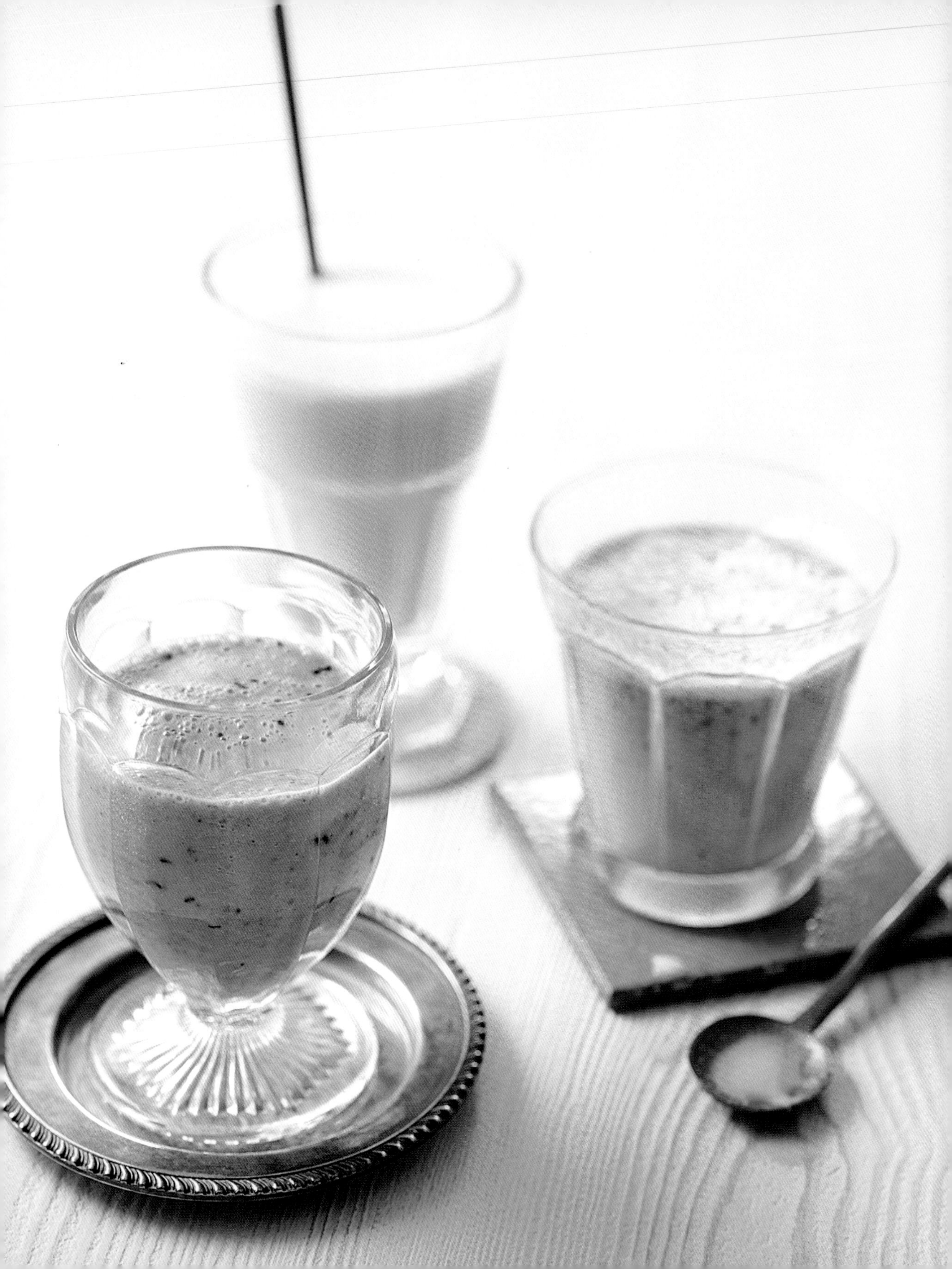

Wide Awake Morning Boost Smoothie

Serves 1

Ingredients

1 green tea bag
3 tablespoons hot water
1 cup water or almond or rice milk
1 scoop BodyBrilliance
3 Brazil nuts
handful of sunflower seeds
handful of pumpkin seeds

Method

1 Brew the green tea bag in the hot water for 3 minutes, then remove the tea bag and stir some honey into the water.

2 Combine the tea-infused water in a blender with the other ingredients, and blend until smooth. Serve immediately.

*it's easy
Healthy habits are a choice that will last you a lifetime. Get started today.

Relaxing Nighttime Smoothie

Serves 1

Ingredients

1 scoop BodySerenity
1 cup vanilla rice milk
handful of ground almonds

Method

Blend all the ingredients together and serve immediately.

The Super Skinny Smoothie

Serves 1

Ingredients

2 Brazil nuts
1 teaspoon chia seeds
1 teaspoon coconut oil
pinch of cinnamon
10 blueberries or raspberries or a combination of both
1 scoop Body Brilliance
1 scoop Ultimate Clean Fiber
½ cup filtered water, rice milk, or almond milk, or equal parts water and milk

Method

Place all the ingredients in a blender and process until smooth. Pour into a tall glass and drink immediately.

*top tip
All Bodyism products are available at bodyism.com and cleanandlean.com.

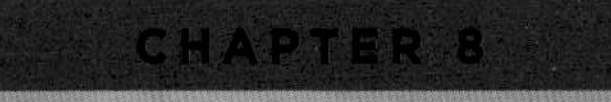
CHAPTER 8

DETOX YOURSELF BEAUTIFUL

THIS CHAPTER WILL REVEAL...

BEAUTY TRICKS TO HELP YOU SLIM DOWN AND LOOK YOUNGER

THE BATH THAT CAN HELP YOU LOSE WEIGHT

HOW CLEAN & LEAN GETS RID OF CELLULITE

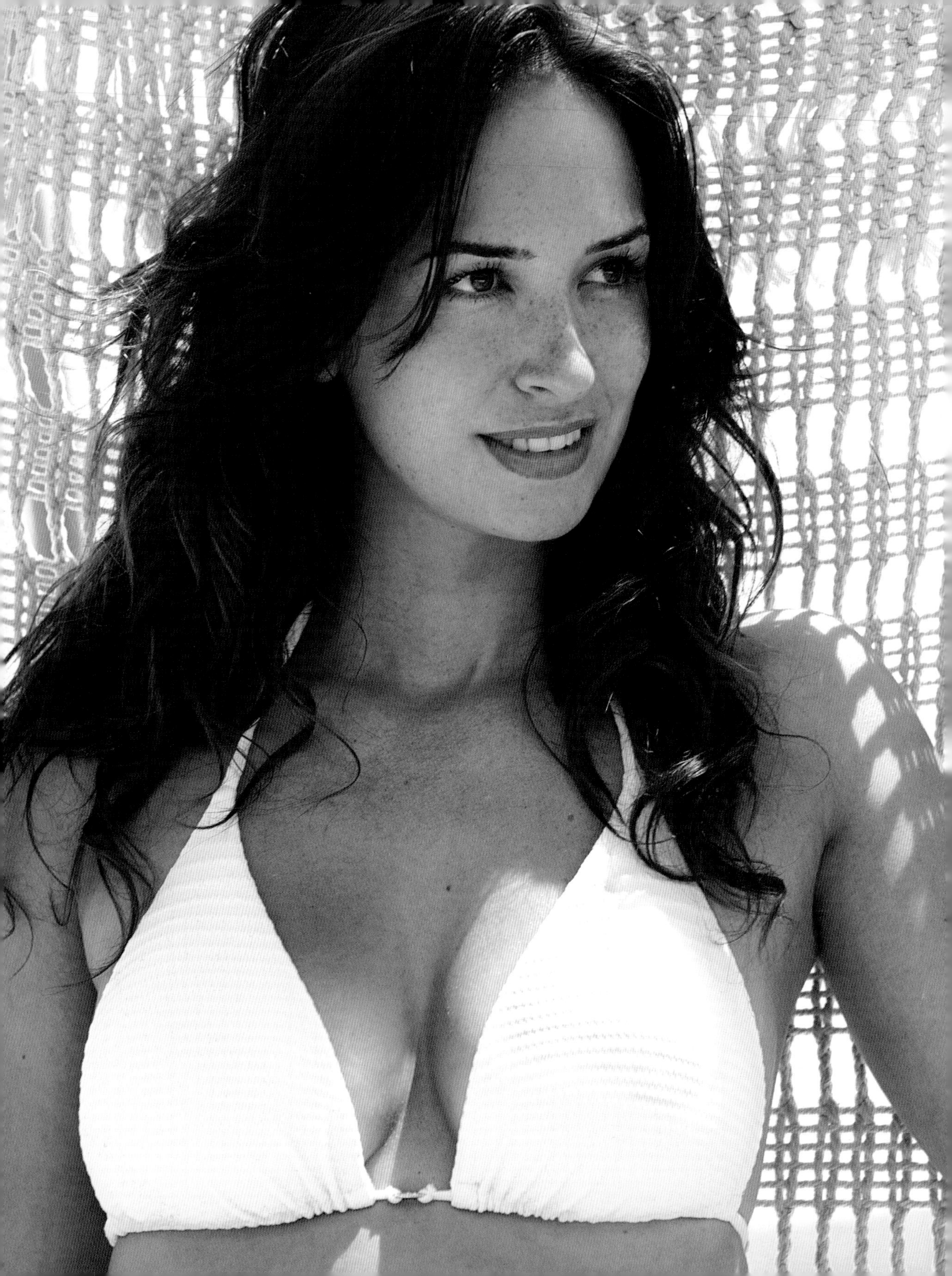

CLEAN & LEAN BEAUTY

The Clean & Lean diet is all about helping your body to shed toxins as effortlessly as possible. This chapter will focus on how detoxing can make you look, as well as feel, better.

Much has been made of the chemicals in beauty products and, while the jury is still out, during the 14-day Kickstart it might be worth switching to organic beauty products. Some studies out there suggest that some of the chemicals in non-organic beauty products end up in your system, though only small amounts—and there's no suggestion as yet that they do any real harm. But as you're detoxing your system anyway, anything that limits the amount of toxins in your body can't be a bad thing (plus lots of the most exclusive, A-list spas worldwide use organic beauty products during their detox regimes).

You don't have to replace your entire bathroom cabinet and make-up bag either, just buy whatever you can afford. If you've given up your frequent trips to the pricey coffee shops and that mid afternoon muffin (which you should have done by now!), then you'll have saved yourself some money to pay for it. The best products to replace are the ones that touch (and therefore sink into) your skin the most—and the ones that you don't wash off. For example, face cream, body lotion, and foundation soak in more because they cover a wider area of skin and because you need to use more of them. So if you can afford it, replace these products rather than those that touch your skin least and you wash off, such as shampoo, conditioner, mascara, eye shadow and lipstick. There are so many fantastic organic beauty ranges out there—go for Neal's Yard (www.nealsyardremedies.com), Organic Pharmacy (www.theorganicpharmacy.com), Liz Earle (us.lizearle.com) and Tisserand (www.tisserand.com).

BEAUTY TRICKS

TO HELP YOU SLIM DOWN AND LOOK YOUNGER

1 Why sugar can make you look old

In Chapter 2 we looked at how sugar can make you fat and ill. But sugar is also potentially one of the biggest aging culprits there is, as it can speed up the appearance of fine lines and wrinkles. When your blood-sugar levels rise, sugar attaches itself to the collagen fibers in your skin. Collagen is the "building brick" of the skin, helping it to stay firm, plump, and youthful looking. When collagen breaks down (usually with age), your skin begins to appear old, wrinkled, and sagging. Too much sugar can break down this "building brick" prematurely, and makes skin less plump and elastic.

2 The Bath That Will Help You to Lose Weight

For a truly lazy way to ditch the toxins, try taking an Epsom salt bath. Many of my model clients swear by this trick. If a client is getting ready for a photo shoot or a holiday, I tell them to soak in Epsom salts in the days leading up to it—the salts are full of magnesium and encourage the body to shed toxins quickly (and remember; these toxins encourage water retention and cling on to fat). The salts also boost your digestion and reduce cellulite. Pour two cupfuls into a hot bath and soak in it for at least 20 minutes up to three times a week. Epsom salts are available online and from pharmacies and health-food shops.

3 The 1-minute body trick to get rid of cellulite

Every single morning, dry body brush yourself all over. Using a decent body brush (they're available in supermarkets and chemists), brush yourself before your shower or bath (not during or after, when your skin will be wet). Start at your feet and brush in light sweeps in the direction of your heart. Go easy on the softer parts of your skin, such as your tummy or breasts. This is quick, cheap, and it'll speed up the whole Clean & Lean process, get your blood pumping and help to reduce the appearance of cellulite. Buy a brush today and get into the habit!

4 How Clean & Lean Gets Rid of Cellulite

Cellulite is a toxic fat that has pushed its way up through the deeper layers of the skin, creating the textured (or "orange peel") appearance on the skin. It's found mainly in fatty areas, like the thighs, bottom, and stomach, but it can also be found on the upper arms.

The more toxic your system is from environmental and dietary pollutants, the more prone to cellulite you'll be. Smoking and living in a busy city toxify your body and encourage dimply thighs. But the worst cellulite offenders are sugar, alcohol, and CRAP (caffeine, refined sugar, alcohol, and processed foods—see Chapter 3).

5 Bodyism Beauty Food

I created this to improve your hair, skin and nails. It's also full of alkalizing supergreens and anti-aging antioxidants. it's the most wonderful thing for your beautiful face and body. As always, you don't have to buy it, it's simply there to make things easier and faster. No hard sell but I'm proud of it and it's amazing. Go to bodyism.com or cleanandlean.com to check it out!

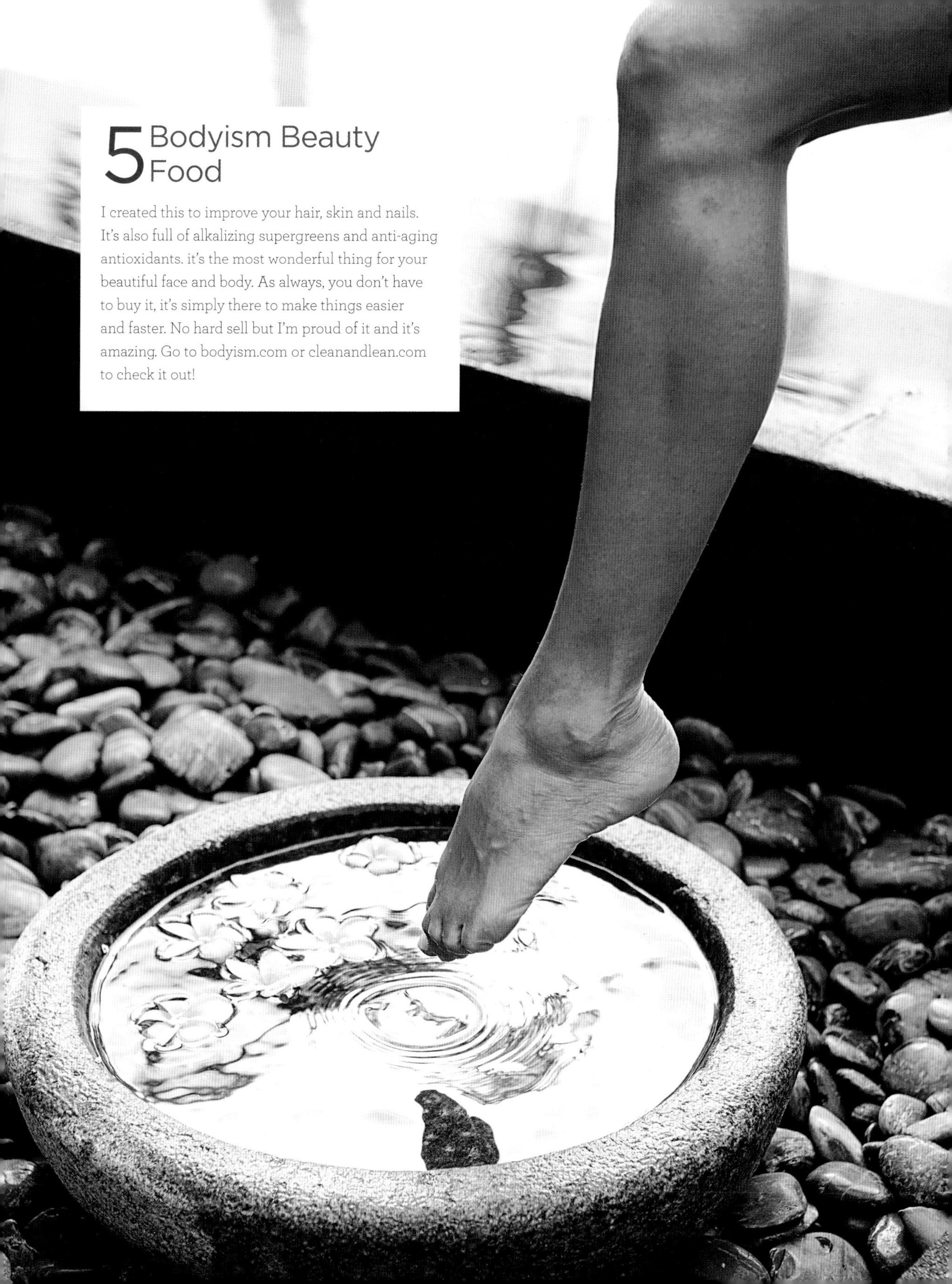

WHAT TO AVOID

The wrong type of water
Yes, really. Tap water can be full of hormones, chemicals, and additives, and is bad for cellulite. Instead, drink filtered or bottled water, ideally from glass bottles. The more pure the water, the less prone to cellulite you will be. Aim for at least 2.5 liters a day.

A toxic environment
As we know, city living causes cellulite. Smog, fumes, and smoking all accumulate and add stress to your body. Avoid these environments wherever possible and try to exercise in nature and away from pollution: for example, walk in the park, not along the road.

Alcohol
Regularly drinking alcohol is a major contributor to cellulite. It's the first thing that needs to go (or at least to be cut back on), if you're serious about getting rid of your cellulite.

Poor circulation
Spending too many hours sitting at a desk isn't good for circulation or burning body fat. Try and get up and stretch, walk around and sneak in some full squats (if you can) every hour or so (see p. 143).

*it's easy

Stick this list on your fridge as a constant reminder, then you won't be tempted to stray.

WHAT TO DO

Eat organically
Try to make sure all your food is organic as it means zero chemicals to toxify your body. This is particularly important when it comes to meat, fish and dairy.

Cut back on coffee
Caffeine makes cellulite worse. Your everyday coffee is a contributor to slowing down your detoxification pathways including your liver (the main organ responsible for detoxing and burning fat). One a day is fine, but any more and you'll increase your chances of getting cellulite.

Be kind to yourself
This is so important! I've said it before and I'll say it again. You DO deserve a happy healthy life, you are important and you do matter. Think as positive as possible, speak kindly about yourself, to yourself and to others.

Ditch the refined carbs
Eating potato chips, fries, breads, and wheat-based breakfast cereals add loads of calories to your diet and contribute to cellulite because of the bad fats these foods contain.

Eat antioxidant-rich fruits
Dark berries all contain high amounts of antioxidants. Also, if you can get your hands on it, the "acai" berry from Brazil contains a higher level of antioxidants than any other known food and is a great cellulite blitzer. I put a teaspoon of freeze-dried acai in my smoothie every morning.

Drink green tea
Green tea contains massive amounts of antioxidants. It's also an excellent alternative to coffee and research at Brisbane's Queensland University also suggests that three cups a day makes it easier to for the body to process sugar and so helps the pounds melt away.

Exercise
Regular exercise helps to promote blood flow and increase your lean muscle mass. The more lean muscle mass you have, the less fat/cellulite you will have!

HOW TO GET CLEAN & LEAN AROUND THE HOME

What applies to your beauty routine also applies to your household cleaning products—there are no firm studies saying that the chemicals in regular bleach, polish or surface cleaners do any harm, but why not go for a slightly less toxic version? Especially during the 14-day Kickstart.

Again, it's about being practical and only swapping what you can afford. Madonna and Gwyneth Paltrow—and lots of other A-listers—use Method cleaning products (well, I imagine they have cleaners that use them but you get my drift!). Method is a brilliant range of chemical-free products using lots of lovely, clean ingredients such as pink grapefruit and fresh lavender. They don't cost much more than regular products, they're very eco-friendly, and you don't even have to wear rubber gloves while using them because they're so natural and toxin-free (methodhome.com).

BAD	BETTER	BEST
Beer—this is packed with sugar, yeast, and alcohol; bad news for cellulite	**Half juice, half water**—if you're serious about getting rid of your cellulite, alcohol is the first thing that must go	**Water**—it flushes your kidneys, liver, and cellulite; drink at least 2.5 liters of filtered water a day
Instant coffee—highly processed and full of toxins that clog your liver; also robs your body of nutrients	**Peppermint tea**—caffeine-free and an excellent digestive aid	**Hot water with 2 or 3 slices of lemon and fresh ginger**—this tonic has a cleansing effect on the liver which helps banish cellulite
White bread—contains very little fiber and protein, the two nutrients that fill you up	**Rye bread**—a wheat-free grain that has loads of fiber	**Super Salad** (see p. 99 for the recipe)—all those greens are a great cellulite-zapper
Soft drinks—packed with sugar, caffeine and empty calories	**Freshly squeezed fruit juice**—all natural sugars with some nutritional value	**A super juice mainly made from greens**—accelerates fat loss and helps cellulite: mix watercress, parsley, spinach, zucchini, green peppers and ginger and drink immediately
Alcopop—contains both alcohol and high amounts of sugar: two ingredients that guarantee cellulite	**Vodka** with mineral water and a squeeze of lime—clean spirit with far fewer calories	**Mineral water with a squeeze of fresh lime**—if you're serious about cellulite then this is the only drink
Potato chips—the thinner the chip is, the fewer nutrients and more bad fats it contains	**Salted, unroasted nuts**—a much better alternative, satisfying your hunger pains with protein as well as your savory craving; maximum one small handful	**Raw, organic, unsalted nuts**—protein in its original raw form, but again, keep the quantity low; one handful only
Ice cream—milk held together with buckets of sugar; most people can't digest dairy properly, lowering their immune system and ability to burn fat	**Natural organic yogurt with almonds**—contains a lot less sugar and the protein from the nuts helps fill you up	**Fresh fruit**—a small handful of berries and half an apple. These are rich in antioxidants and detox your system
French fries—high starch, very little fiber coated in transfats (the worst fats of all)	**Baked potato**—much more fibrous and filling than fries or potato wedges; even better with some protein like chicken or tuna	**Steamed vegetables**—adding a sliver of organic butter helps release the minerals in the vegetables, as well as helping to fill you up

BAD	BETTER	BEST
Salad dressing—ultra-high in bad fats and sugars; don't be fooled by low-fat versions or healthy-looking labels, these are just full of salt and fake ingredients	**Extra-virgin olive oil**—contains essential fatty acids; a "good" fat that helps your body burn calories	**Olives**—a great source of the omega 3 and 6 essential fatty acids that help kick fat out of your fat cells and into your bloodstream, where they can be burned off more easily, and with more fiber than oil
Muesli/granola bars—these masquerade as healthy but are full of sugar	**Dried fruit and nuts**—contain fruit sugars and some complete protein; not a bad snack!	**Raw vegetables**—broccoli, celery, carrots, cucumber, and cauliflower are jam packed with nutrients and have very few calories
Cakes—loaded with sugar, wheat, yeast, and bad fats	**Muffin** from health-food shop—contains fiber and fewer bad fats	**Fruit and nuts**—contain fruit sugars and some complete protein
Chocolate bar—convenient, pocket-sized fat bomb	**Fruit and nuts**—contain fruit sugars and some complete protein	**Raw cucumber with some avocado**—avocado is high in monounsaturated fat. This snack will fill you up and leave you energized without the inevitable sugar crash of chocolate
Croissant—zero fiber and soaked in bad fats; probably the worst breakfast known to cellulite	**Muffin from health-food shops**—contains fiber and fewer bad fats	**Raw vegetables with just a little organic hummus**—loads of fiber, vitamins, and minerals
Cookies—empty calories, full of salt, sugar, and the bad fats lead to cellulite	**Oatcake with nut butter**—wheat-free, contains some fiber, protein, and good fats	**Rice cake with turkey and avocado**—the perfect blend of proteins, carbs, and good fats
Pasta dish, such as lasagne—packed with bad fats and coated with calories from the cheese and cheese sauce	**Steak and salad**—a simple dish containing all the nutrients you need	**Organic steak and Super Salad** (see p. 98)—organic meat contains fewer toxins, and zero hormones; choose a lean cut and serve with a brightly colored salad
Burger and fries—nutritionally very poor, the bread is often so sugary it's classified as a pastry and sometimes there's not real potato in the fries	**Burger without the bun and salad**—breadless means fewer empty carbs and more room for a fresh salad	**Lean beef stir-fry with loads of vegetables**—quick and delicious; feeds your muscles and burns your fat
Fried chicken—usually poor-quality meat surrounded by a layer of lard!	**Barbecued chicken with salad**—better-quality protein; just take off the skin to avoid cellulite	**Skinless turkey breast with a brightly colored salad**—turkey is lean meat packed with protein

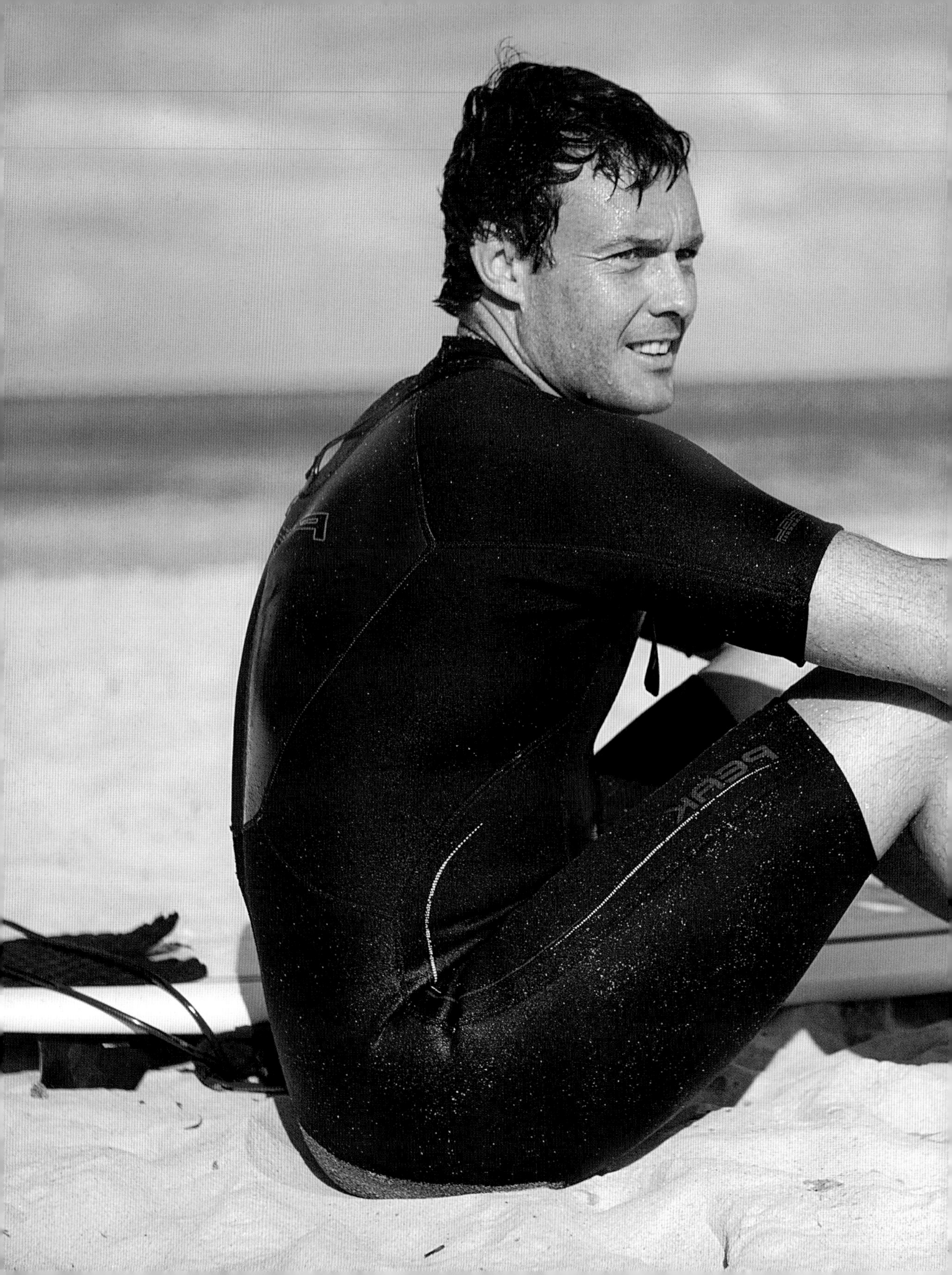
PEAK

CHAPTER 9

YOUR EASY EXERCISE PLAN

THIS CHAPTER WILL REVEAL...

THE 12-MINUTE WORKOUT TO DO EVERY DAY

HOW IMPROVING YOUR POSTURE MAKES YOU SLIMMER

WHY EXERCISE MAKES YOU LOOK YOUNGER

YOUR WORKOUTS

These custom workouts have been created to sculpt a variety of muscles, while burning fat and creating a beautiful posture.

1 The programs are designed in a circuit format. Having used this method to train our clients at Bodyism, we know it works.

2 To get the best from your workout it's important to perform each circuit in the order specified, while following the recommended number of sets.

3 Perform each exercise immediately one after the other, but be sure to take the indicated rest period after each exercise.

4 Simply follow each move slowly and with control. If you experience any pain, stop immediately.

5 Begin with the 12-minute program. Perform this phase three times a week on non-consecutive days until you can complete all the repetitions in the workout. Then progress to the 18-minute, 23-minute and 25-minute program.

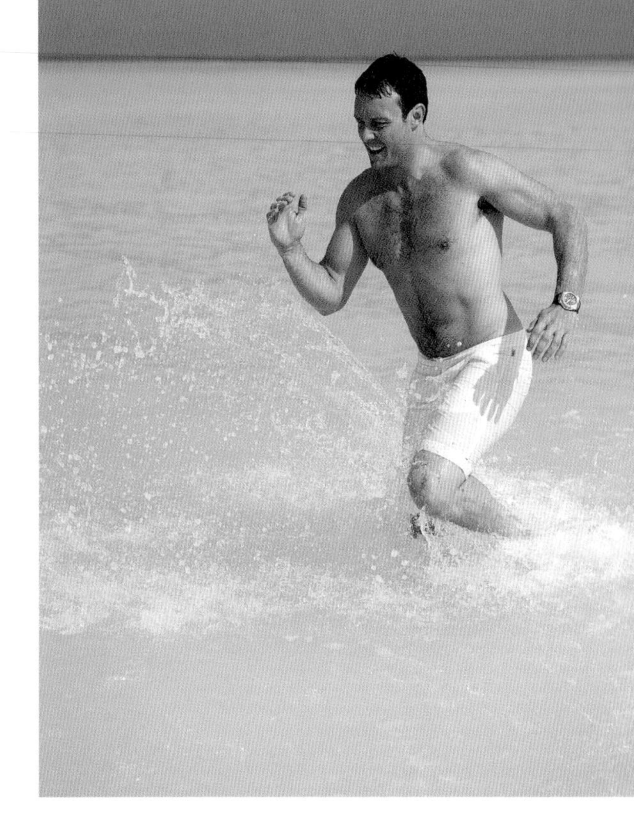

4-WEEK WORKOUT BLUEPRINT

WEEK 1	WEEK 2	WEEK 3	WEEK 4
Monday 12-minute program	**Monday** 18-minute program	**Monday** 23-minute program	**Monday** 25-minute program
Wednesday 12-minute program	**Wednesday** 18-minute program	**Wednesday** 23-minute program	**Wednesday** 25-minute program
Friday 12-minute program	**Friday** 18-minute program	**Friday** 23-minute program	**Friday** 25-minute program

THE PROGRAMS

12-MINUTE

Movement prep

✳ Lying 90 – 90 Stretch (p. 138) 1 x 10 reps each side/ 15-second rest

✳ Hamstring Stretch (p. 136) 1 x 10 reps each side/ 15-second rest

Pre-hab

✳ Hip Extension (p. 141) 1 x 10 reps/ 30-second rest

✳ Lying Y (p. 144) 1 x 10 reps/ 30-second rest

✳ Mini Band Single Knee External Rotation (p. 142) 1 x 10 reps each leg/ 30-second rest

Main workout

✳ Split Squat (p. 147) 1 x 10 reps each leg/ 30-second rest

✳ Push Up From Knees (p. 147) 1 x 10 reps/ 30-second rest

✳ The Squat (p. 88) 1 x 10 reps/ 30-second rest

✳ Standing Y's (p. 149) 1 x 10 reps/ 60-second rest

✳ The Plank (p. 150) 1 x 15-second hold/ 30-second rest

Regeneration

✳ The Skinny Stretch (p. 164) 1 x 5 reps each side

18-MINUTE

Movement prep

✳ Lying 90 – 90 Stretch (p. 138) 1 x 10 reps each side/ 15-second rest

✳ Hamstring Stretch (p. 136) 1 x 10 reps each side/ 30-second rest

Pre-hab

✳ Single Leg Hip Extension (p. 141) 2 x 10 reps each leg/ 30-second rest

✳ Lying T (p. 144) 2 x 10 reps/ 30-second rest

✳ Band Walking (p. 143) 2 x 10 reps each way/ 60-second rest then repeat the circuit

Main workout

✳ Reverse Dynamic Lunge (p. 151) 2 x 10 reps each leg/ 30-second rest

✳ Push Up from Feet (p. 152) 2 x 10 reps/ 30-second rest

✳ The Squat (p. 88) 2 x 10 reps/ 30-second rest

✳ Weighted T (p. 153) 2 x 10 reps/ 60-second rest then repeat the circuit

✳ The Plank (p. 150) 2 x 30-second holds/ 30-second rest then repeat

Regeneration

✳ The Skinny Stretch (p. 164) 1 x 5 reps each side

22-MINUTE

Movement prep

✳ Lying 90 – 90 Stretch (p. 138) 1 x 10 reps each side/ 15-second rest

✳ Hamstring Stretch (p. 136) 1 x 10 reps each side/ 30-second rest

Pre-hab

✳ Hip Extension (p. 141) 2 x 15 reps/ 15-second rest

✳ Standing Y (p. 149) 2 x 15 reps/ 15-second rest

✳ Mini Band Single Knee External Rotation (p. 142) 2 x 15 reps each leg/ 60-second rest then repeat the circuit

Main workout

✳ Push Press (p. 154) 2 x 15 reps/ 30-second rest

✳ Dynamic Lunge with Rotation (p. 155) 2 x 15 reps each leg/ 30-second rest

✳ Single Leg Push Up (p. 88) 2 x 10 reps/ 30-second rest

✳ Static Lunge with Bicep curl (p. 157) 2 x 10 reps each leg/ 30-second rest

✳ Weighted Y (p. 153) 2 x 15 reps/ 60-second rest then repeat the circuit

✳ Single Leg Plank (p. 158) 2 x 30-second holds/ 30-second rest then repeat

✳ Burpie (p. 159) 2 x 30 reps/ 60-second rest then repeat

Regeneration

✳ The Skinny Stretch (p. 164) 1 x 5 reps each side

25-MINUTE

Movement prep

✳ Lying 90 – 90 Stretch (p. 138) 1 x 10 reps each side/ 15-second rest

✳ Hamstring Stretch (p. 136) 1 x 10 reps each side/ 30-second rest

Pre-hab

✳ Single Leg Hip Extension (p. 141) 2 x 15 reps each leg/ 30-second rest

✳ Standing T (p. 145) 2 x 15 reps/ 15-second rest

✳ Band Walking (p. 143) 2 x 15 reps each way/ 60-second rest then repeat the circuit

Main workout

✳ Single Leg Squat (p. 160) 2 x 10 reps each leg/ 30-second rest

✳ Push Up with Feet Elevated (p. 161) 2 x 10 reps/ 30-second rest

✳ Lunge with Shoulder Press (p. 88) 2 x 10 reps/ 30-second rest

✳ Weighted T (p. 153) 2 x 10 reps/ 30-second rest

✳ Single Leg Plank (p. 158) 2 x 30-second holds/ 30-second rest then repeat

✳ Burpie (p. 159) 2 x 1 minute/ 90-second rest then repeat the circuit

Regeneration

✳ The Skinny Stretch (p. 164) 1 x 5 reps each side

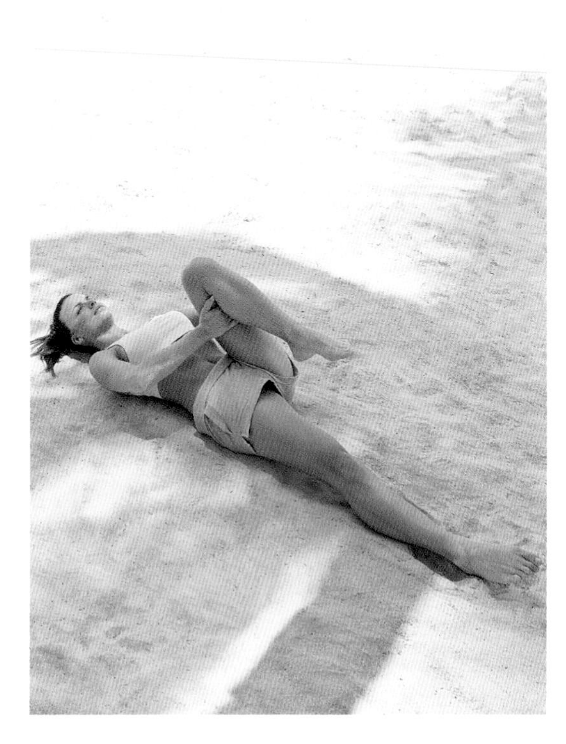

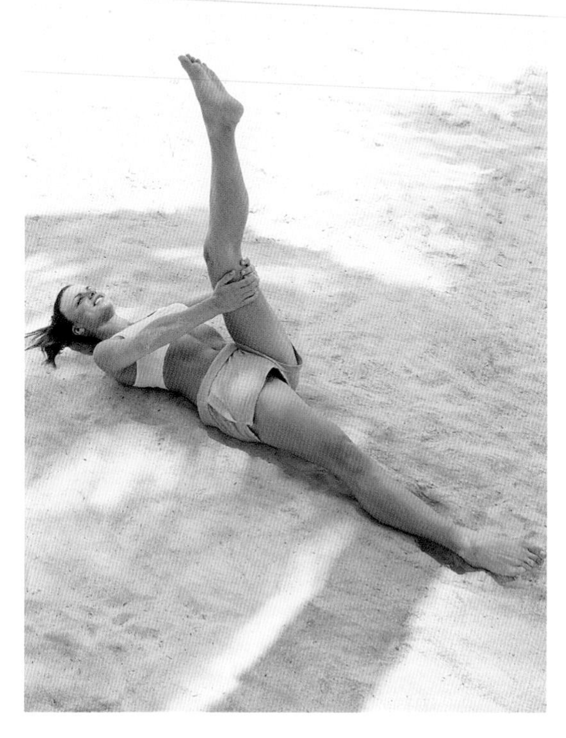

Lying Hamstring Stretch

How to do it

1 Start by lying on your back. Place your hands behind your bent knee, then slowly lift your leg ensuring that it remains straight and your toes are pointing towards your head. The other leg should remain straight and in contact with the floor at all times, to ensure your hips stay flat.

2 Once you feel a stretch in the hamstring, hold for 3–5 seconds.

3 After the first sequence is complete; slowly turn the toe out and hold for 3–5 seconds. Then turn the toe in and switch legs.

4 If you feel pain in your lower back roll a towel and place it under your lower back for support.

*top tip

This stretch is great for loosening up tight hamstrings. By alternating the foot position it allows all the different areas of the muscle to be stretched.

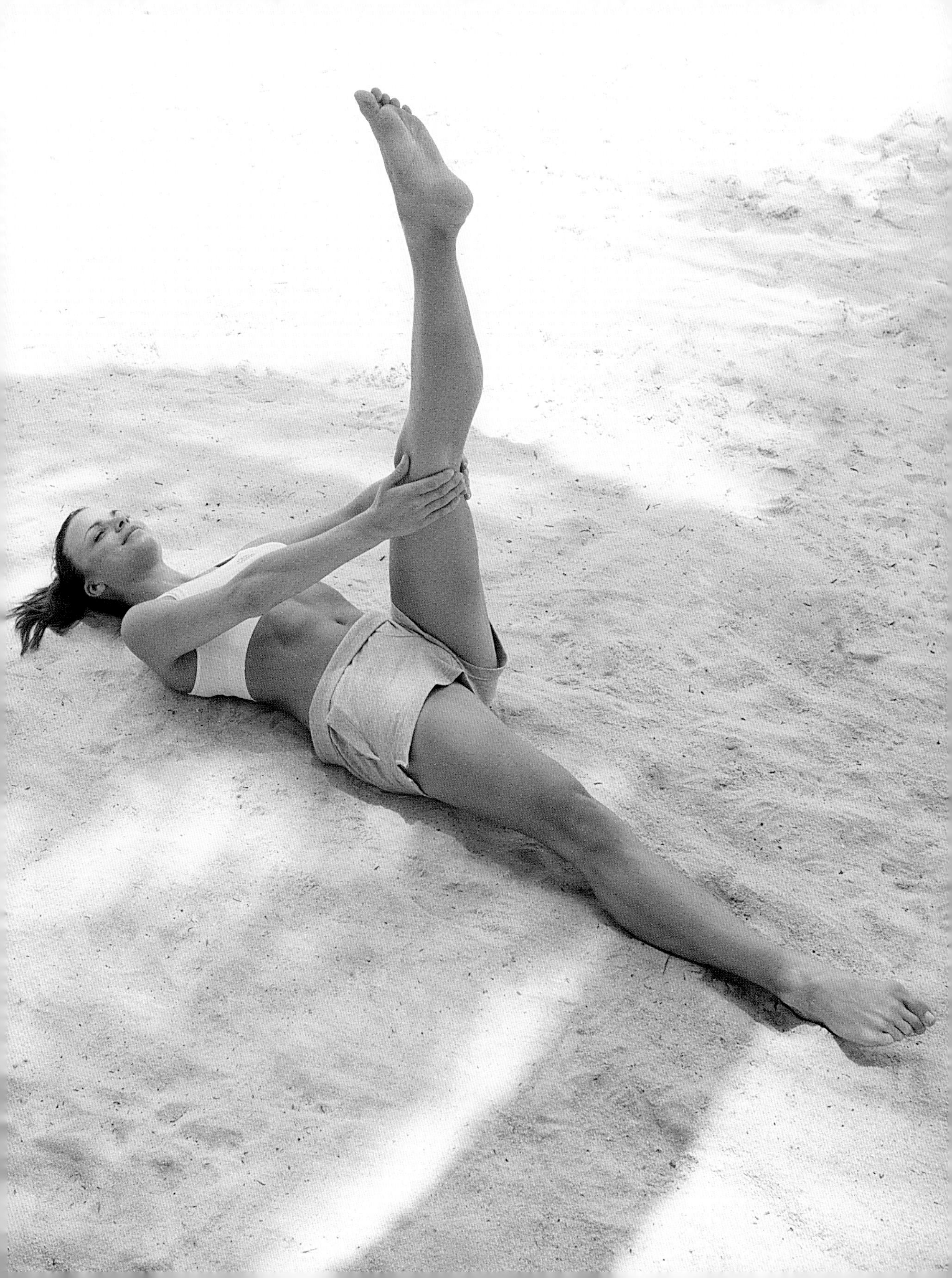

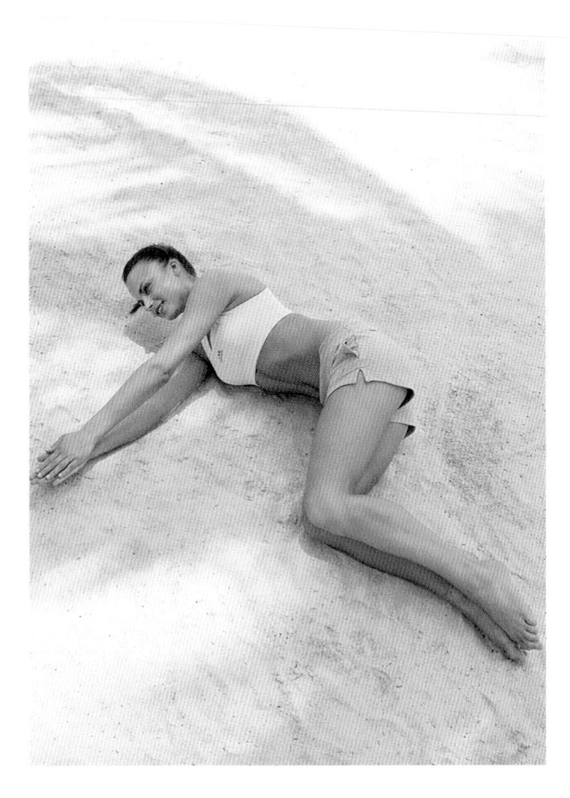

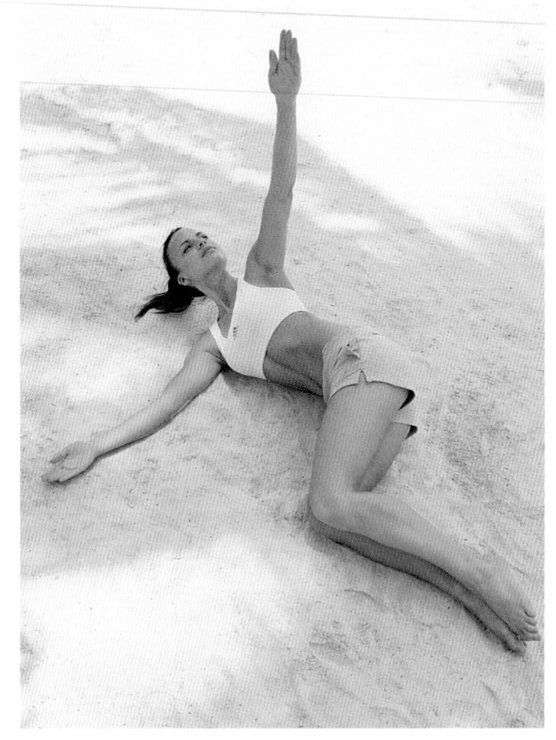

Lying 90-90 Stretch

How to do it

1 Lie on your side with your legs bent at a 90-degree angle, with your arms out straight in front of you.
2 Slowly rotate one arm up and then towards the opposite side keeping your knees squeezed together.

*top tip

This is great for upper body mobility and loosening you up.

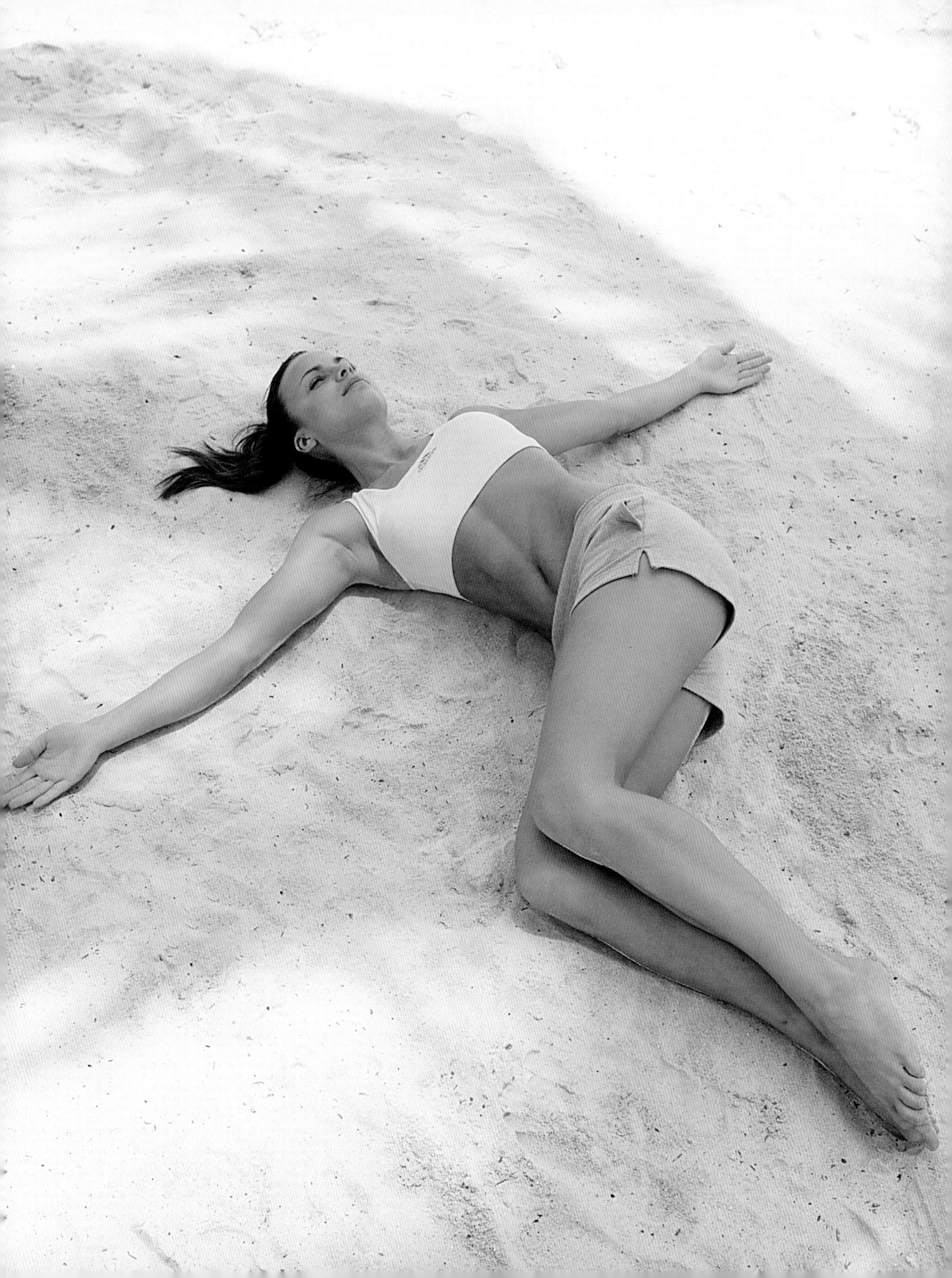

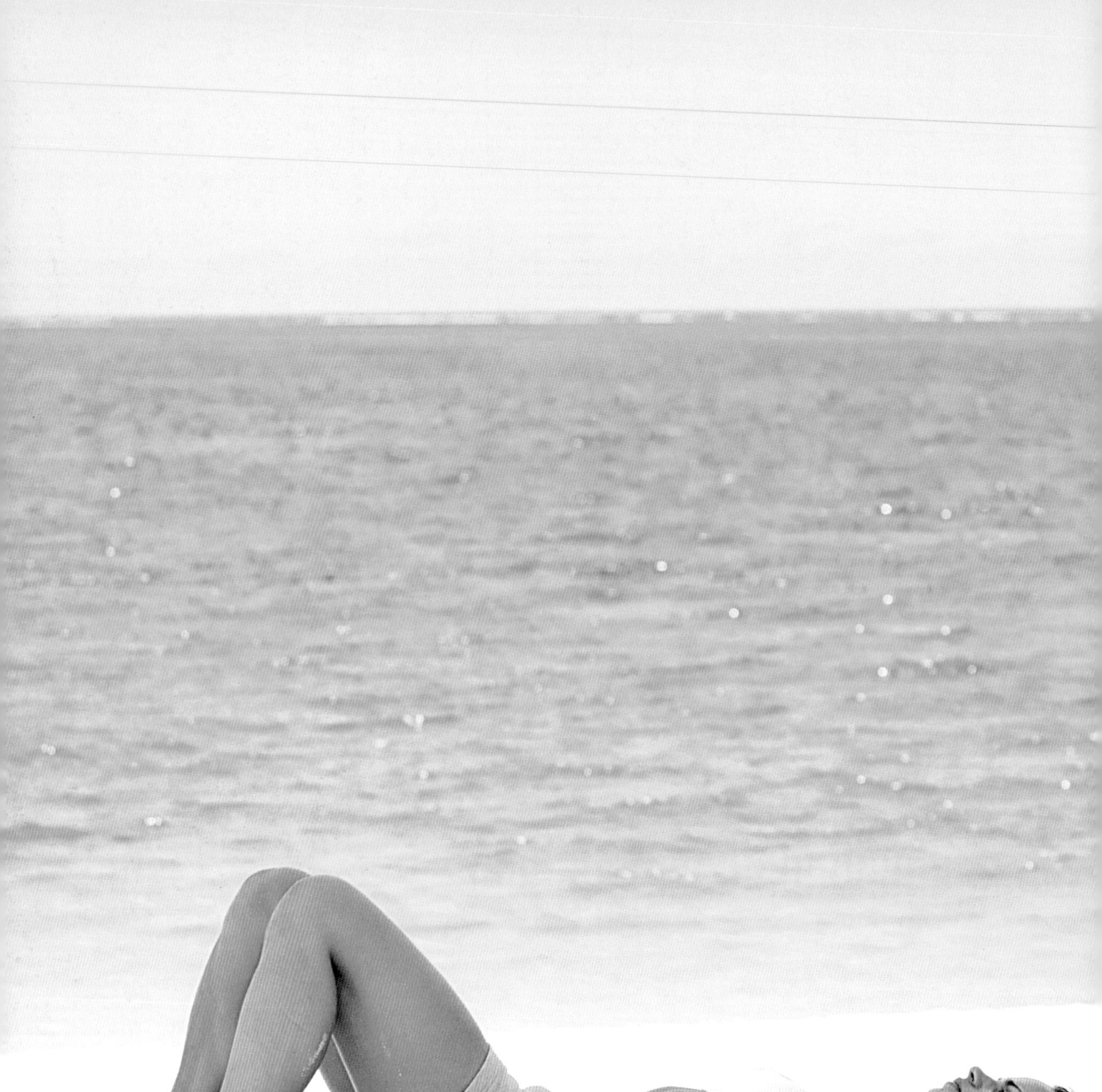

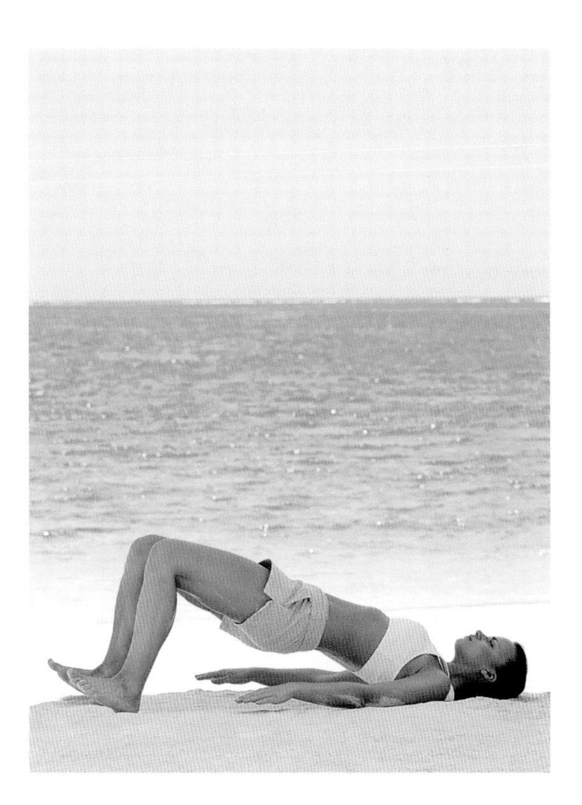

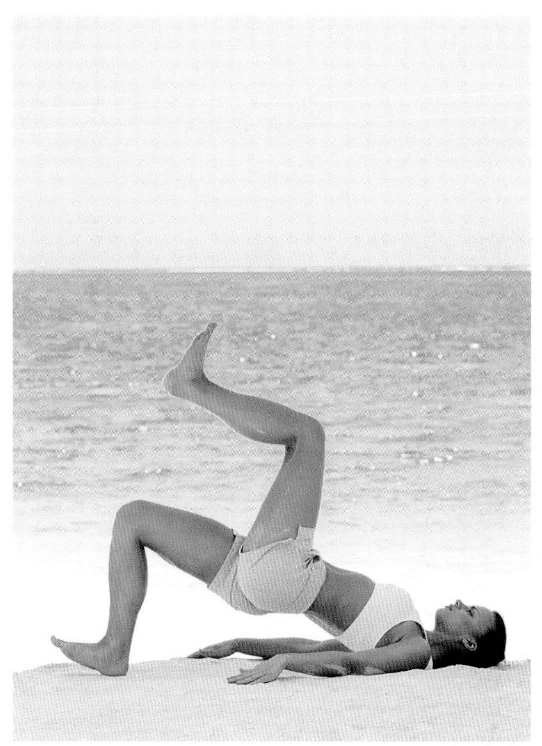

Hip Extension

1 Lay on your back with your knees bent and heels on the ground and your toes pointing up.
2 Lift your hips off the ground, not letting your bottom touch the ground on the way down.

Single Leg Hip Extension

1 With your hips still lifted (your body should be in a straight line off the floor), raise one knee up and lower it.
2 Repeat the same thing with the other knee lifted.

*it's easy

This is great for your bottom and lower back.

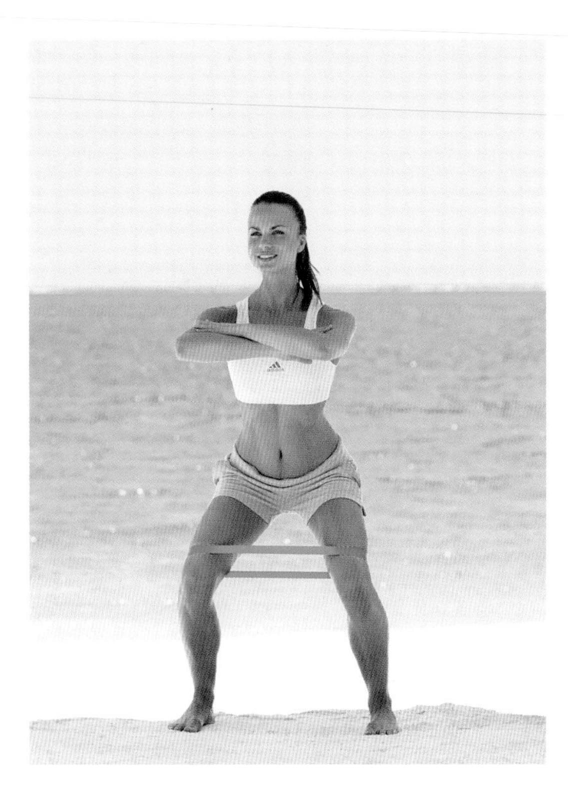

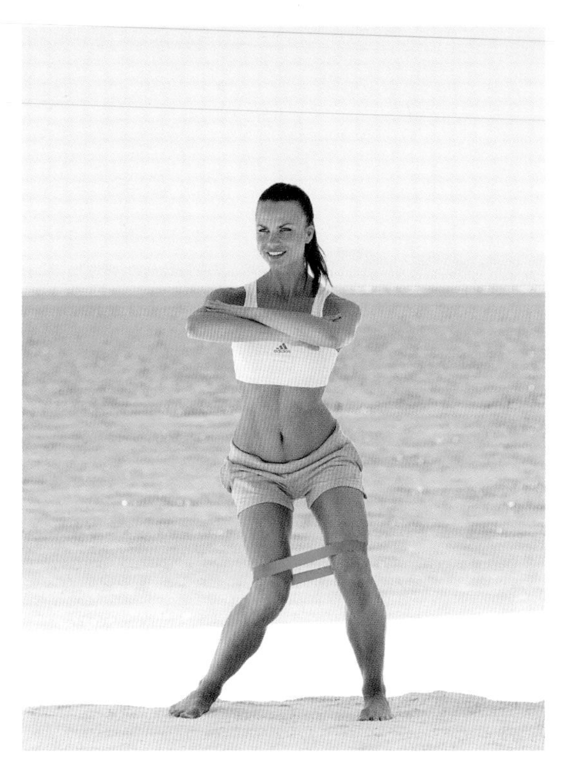

External Knee Rotation with Bodyism Band

How to do it

1 Put the band around your knees.
2 Get into a squat position and bring one knee in towards the other knee.
3 Try to keep the rest of the body still.
4 Repeat with the other knee.

*top tip

This switches on your hip and thigh muscles and works your core (stomach) muscles.

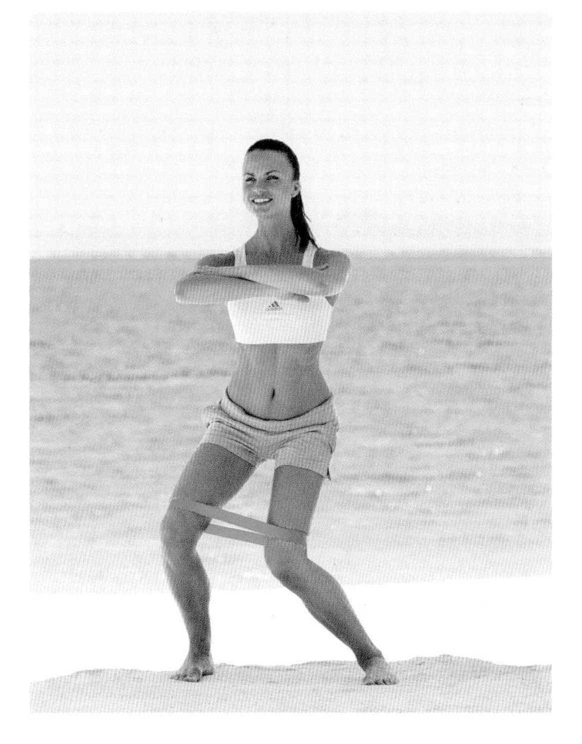

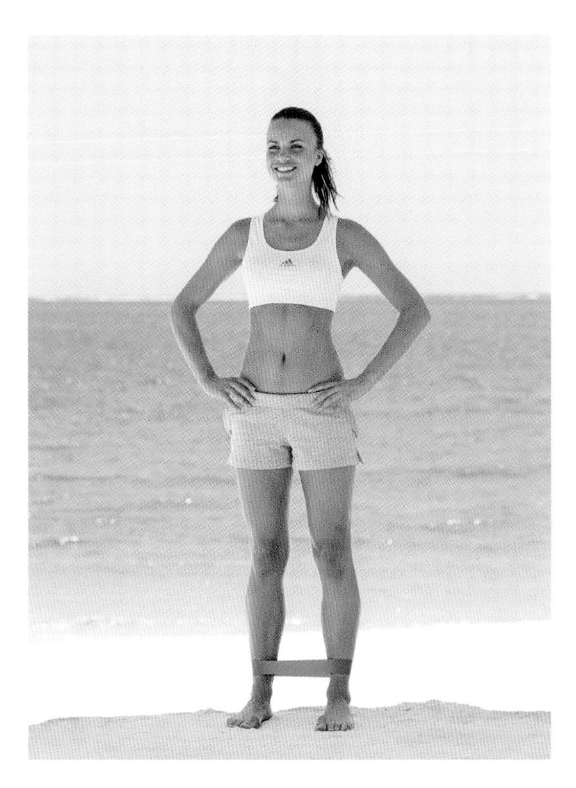

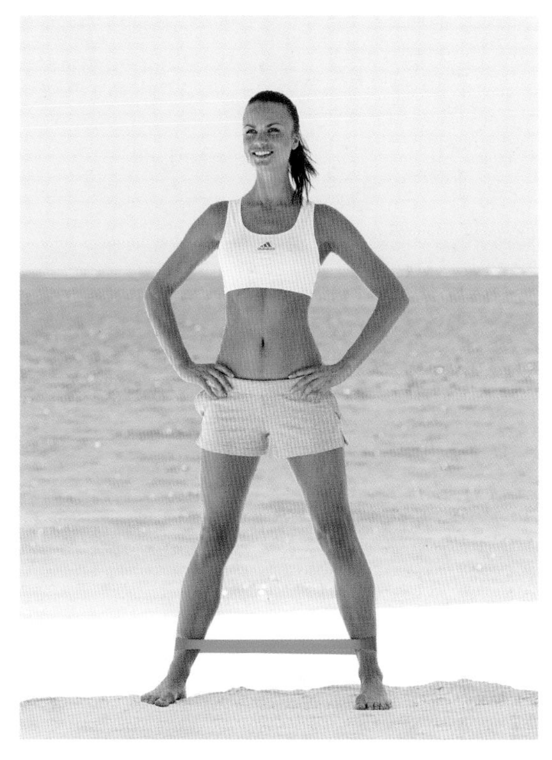

Exercise Band Walking

How to do it

1 Put the band around your ankles and walk slowly, keeping tension in the band. At all times keep the upper body as still as possible.

2 Now place the band above the knees, get into a squat position and walk again.

*top tip

This lifts your bottom like nothing else. It helps stabilize the knee, hip, and ankle joints.

*equipment

You need an exercise band—you can buy these at most sports shops or online at www.bodyism.com. If you don't want to buy one, just do 20 squats instead of the exercises at left. (See page 148 for how to do a squat.)

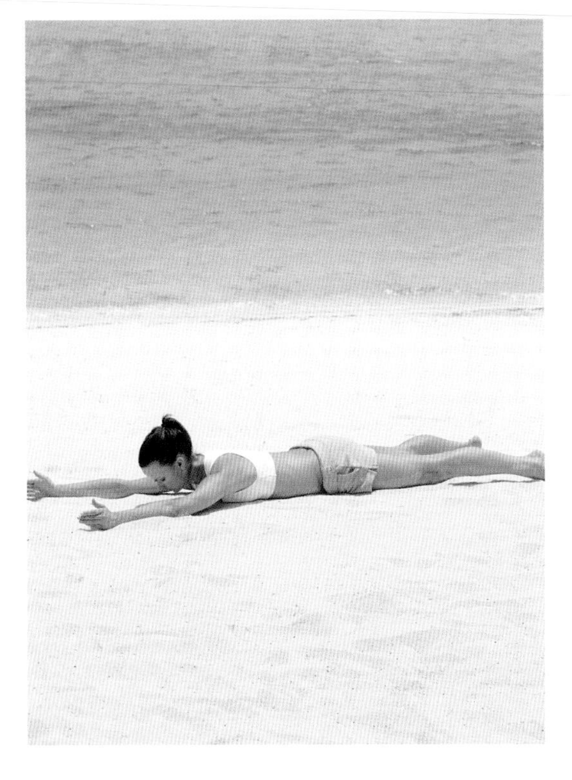

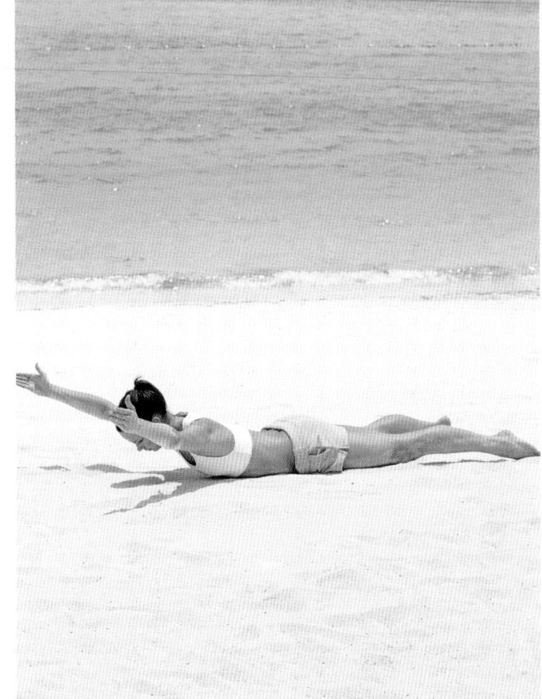

The Lying Y & T Move

How to do The Y

1 Lie on your stomach with your arms up and out above your head so your whole body is making a "Y" shape.

2 Slowly draw your shoulder blades together and lift your arms off the floor.

How to do The T

1 Lie on your stomach with your arms extended out to the side so your whole body is making a "T" shape.

2 Slowly draw your shoulder blades together and lift your arms off the floor.

*top tip

This move switches on all the postural muscles of the upper back, helping you stand straighter and longer. Good posture can take 11 lbs off someone when they stand straight.

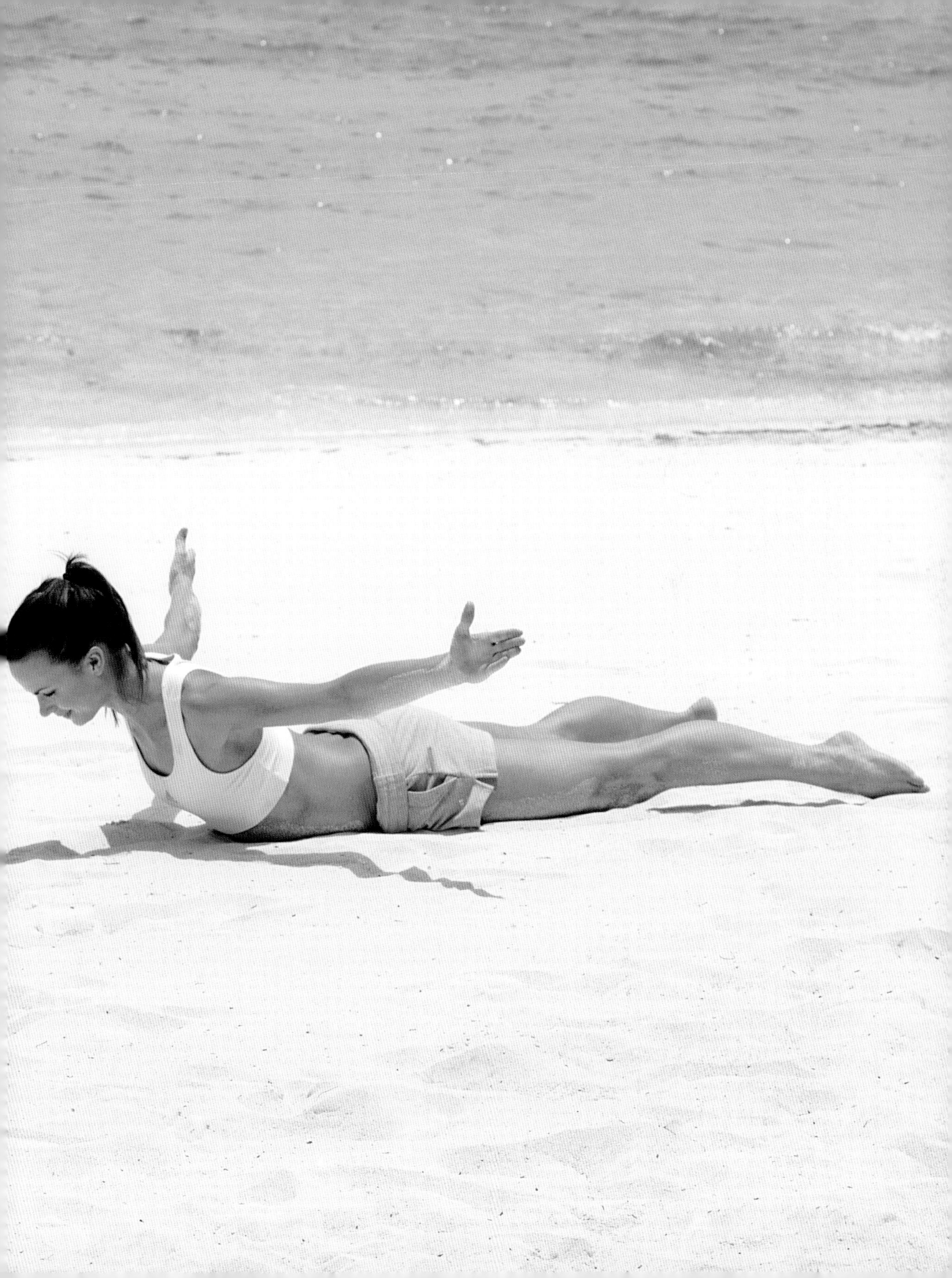

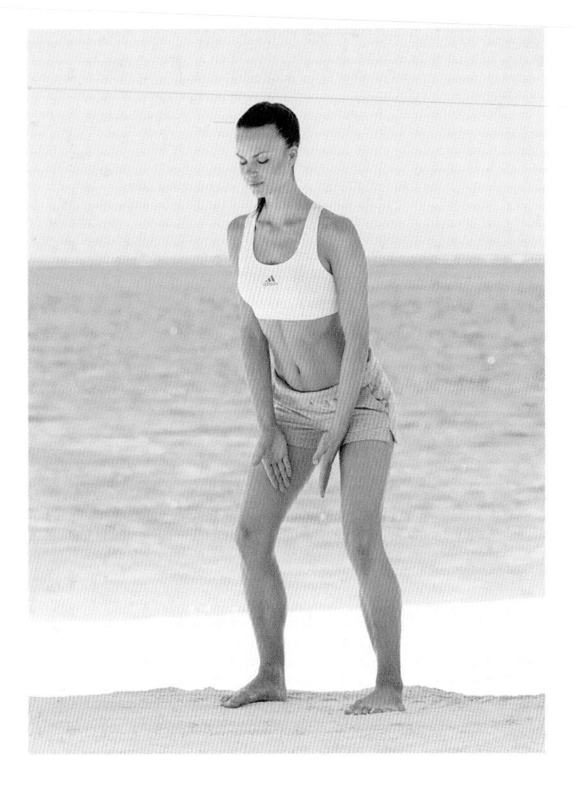

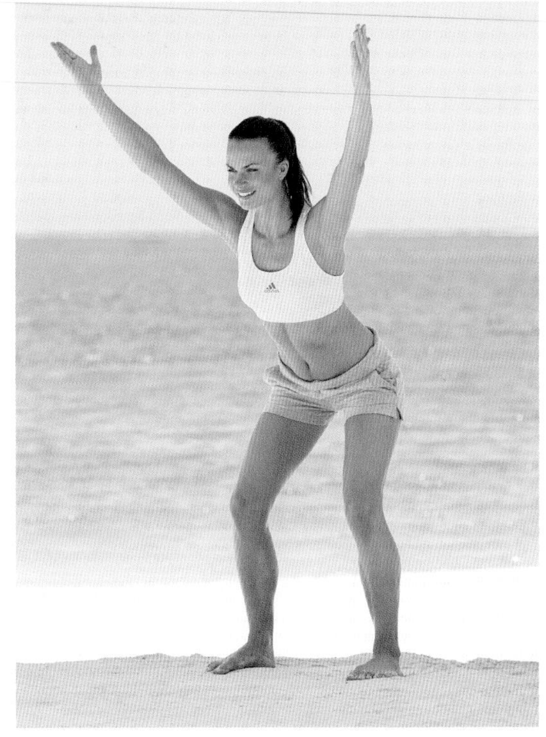

Standing Y + T

How to do it

1 Bend your legs and stick your bottom out.

2 Keep your back and head all in a straight line, shoulders down, and back and keep the tummy tight.

3 Bring both arms alongside your ears in a straight line making a "Y."

4 Everything is the same with the "T" but bend down a little further and bring your arms to the side making a "T."

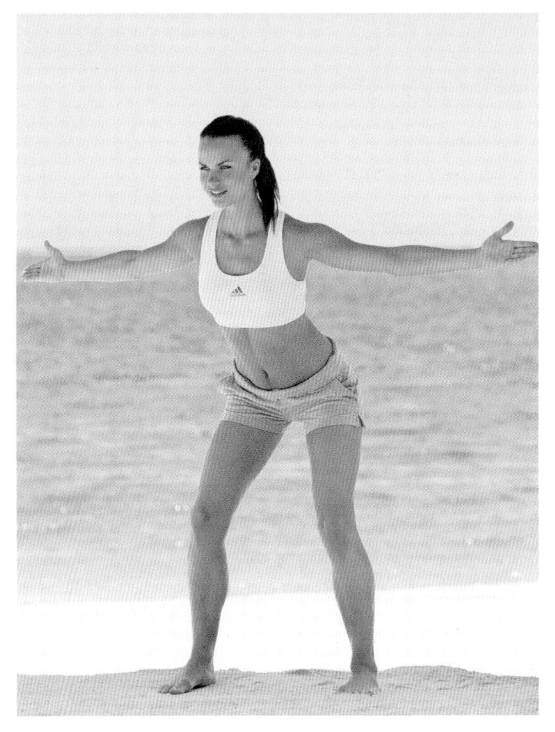

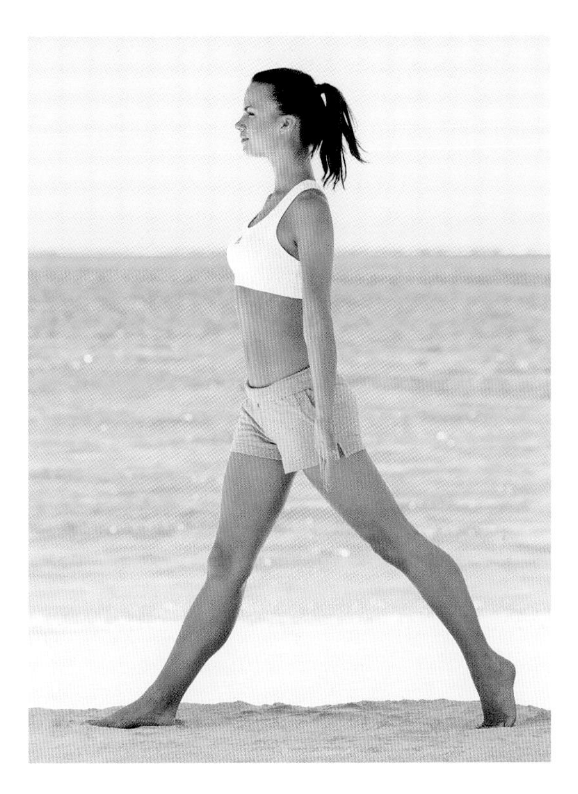

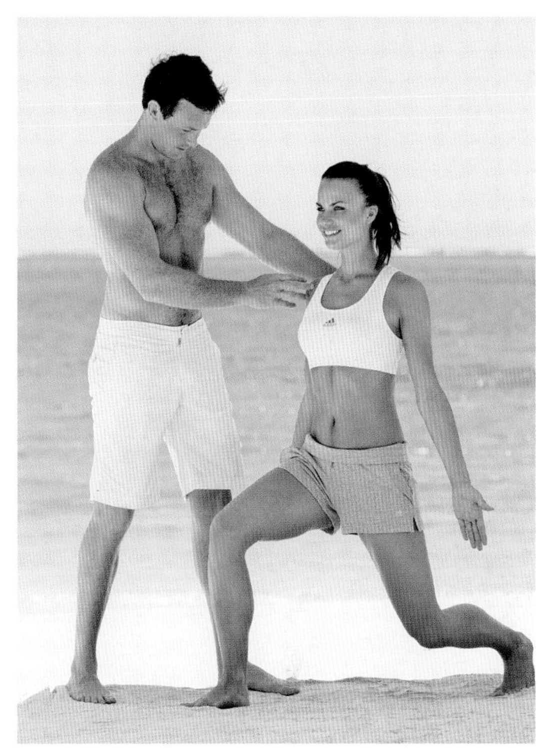

Split Squat

How to do it

1 Stand with perfect posture with your palms facing out.
2 Both feet should face forwards.
3 Contract your stomach muscles.
4 Feet should be hip-width apart.
5 Position your feet, as shown top left, with straight front shin.
6 Lower your body by bending your back knee, as shown right. The back knee should just touch the floor.
7 Push up by pushing off the heel of the front foot. Repeat on the other leg.

*top tip

Great for your butt, hips and thighs! This move uses several muscles so it burns loads of fat. And when you do it right, it will improve your posture.

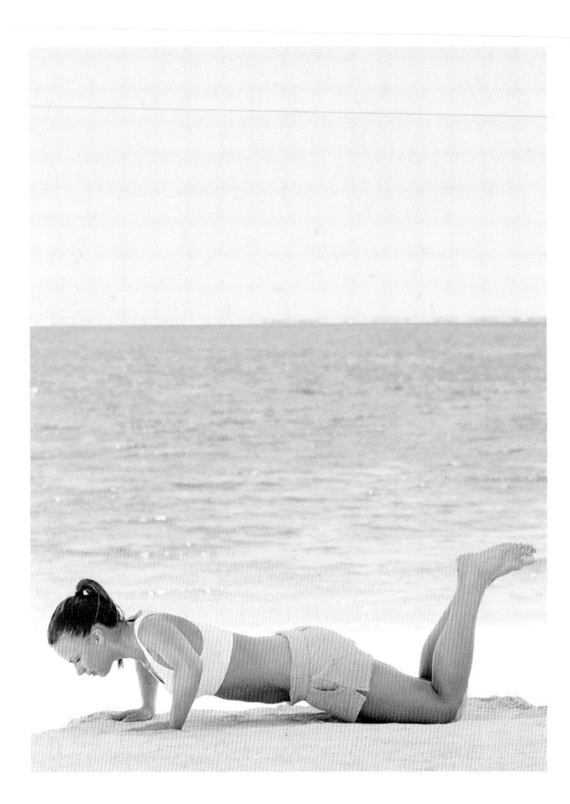

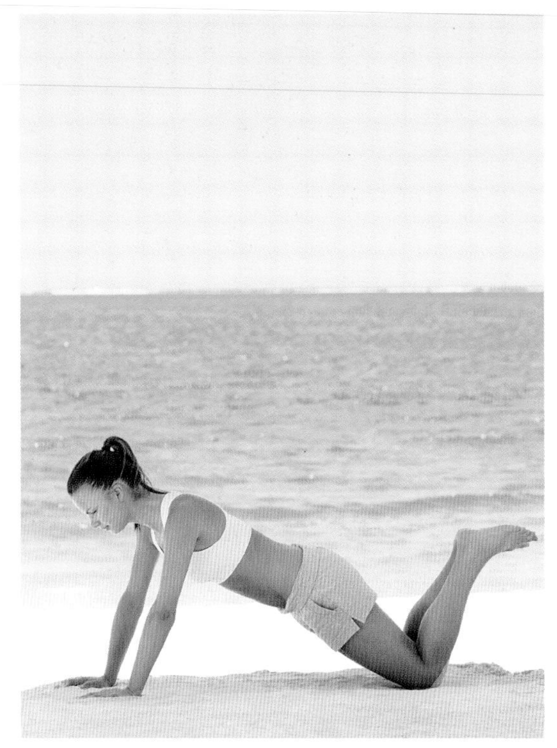

Push Up from Knees

*top tip

The push up strengthens your upper body and works your abdominals, plus it's a great way to tone your arms and chest.

How to do it

1 Place your knees on the ground.
2 Set your hands one and a half shoulder widths apart and in line with your nipples, NOT your shoulders.
3 Keep your ears, shoulders and hips in alignment.
4 Contract your stomach muscles.
5 Lower yourself so your nose almost touches the ground, keeping your body straight, then lift back up to the start position.
6 Remember to keep your head up and belly button drawn in.
7 Breathe out as you push up to start position, and breathe in as you lower yourself down.

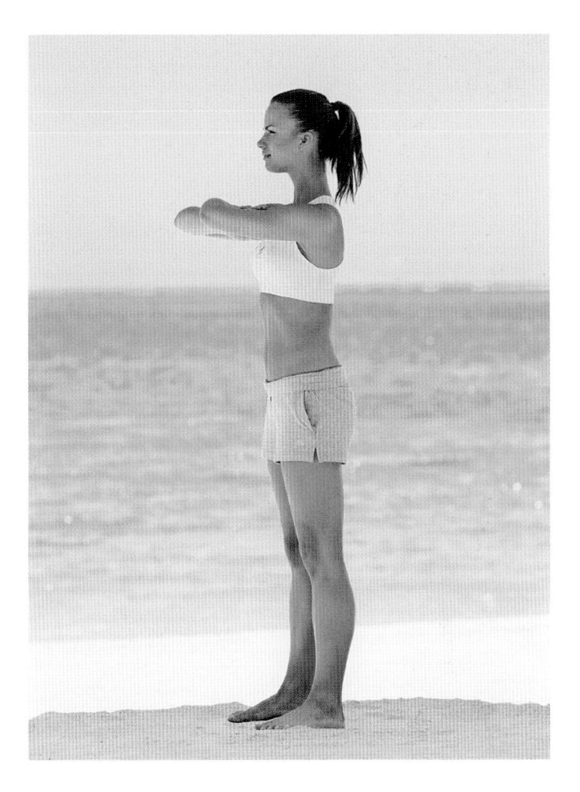

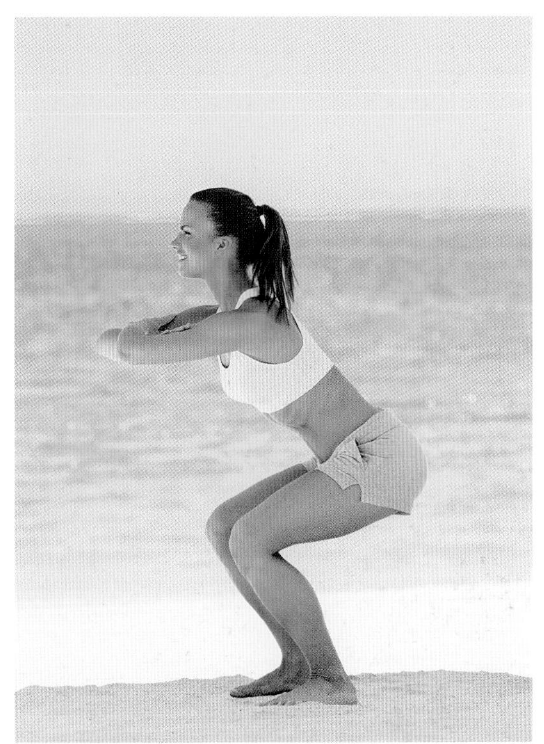

The Squat

How to do it

1 Contract your stomach muscles.
2 Take a comfortable stance, keeping your feet shoulder-width apart, wider if necessary.
3 Cross your arms and hold them parallel to the floor.
4 Point your toes out slightly and make sure your knees stay aligned with your second toe, and DO NOT fall forwards or inwards when squatting. Keep your weight in your heel.
5 Keeping your heels on the floor, lower yourself until your thighs are parallel with the floor. Stick your butt out.
6 Go as low as you comfortably can while maintaining perfect posture (straight back, ears over shoulders).
7 Push up through your heels and return to a standing position.

*top tip

This sculpts your butt, stomach and legs, it burns lots of fat and even improves your posture.

The Plank

How to do it

1 Lie face down on the floor with forearms and elbows touching the floor, hips and legs on the ground.

2 Raise your hips and set the core, keeping your head aligned with your upper back and hips. Imagine a straight line from your head to your ankles.

*top tip

Helping you towards a flatter stomach, the plank is also great for your back. This is a fantastic way to work your abs without the neck strain of a sit-up!

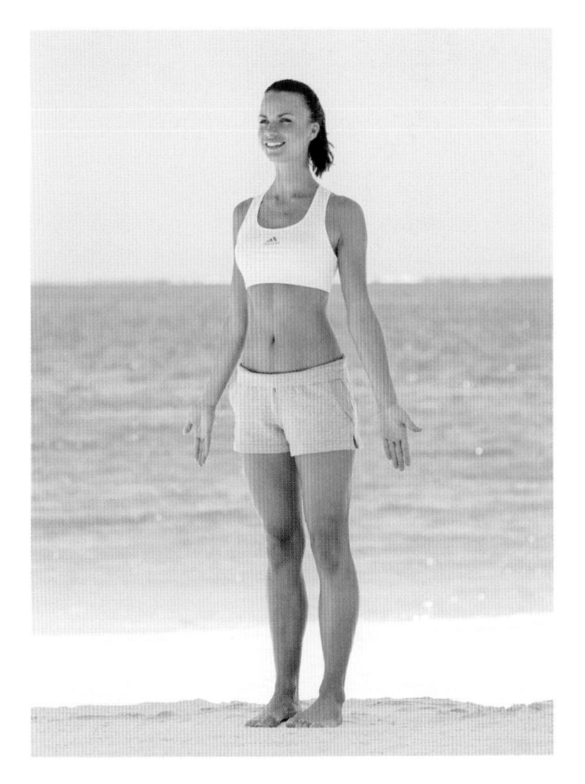

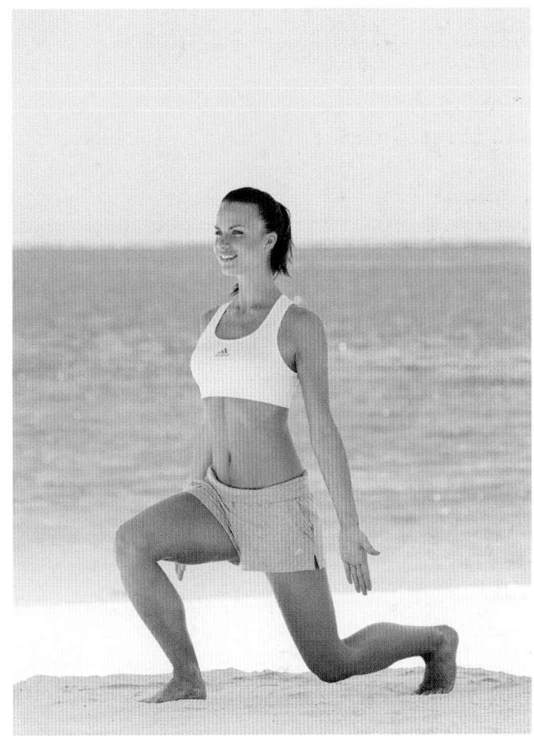

Reverse Dynamic Lunge

How to do it

1 Stand up with perfect posture (see Split Squat, as before) with palms facing outwards.
2 Both feet should face out.
3 Set the core.
4 Your feet should be hip-width apart.
5 Step backwards as shown. Your front shin should be straight and perpendicular to the floor.
6 Push up with the front legs returning to a standing position.

*it's easy
This burns even more fat than the Split Squat and is great for your butt, hips, and thighs.

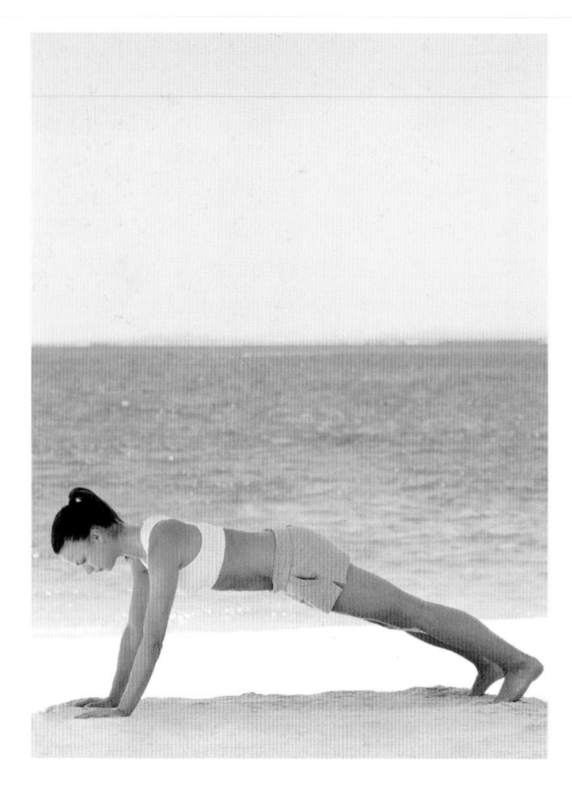

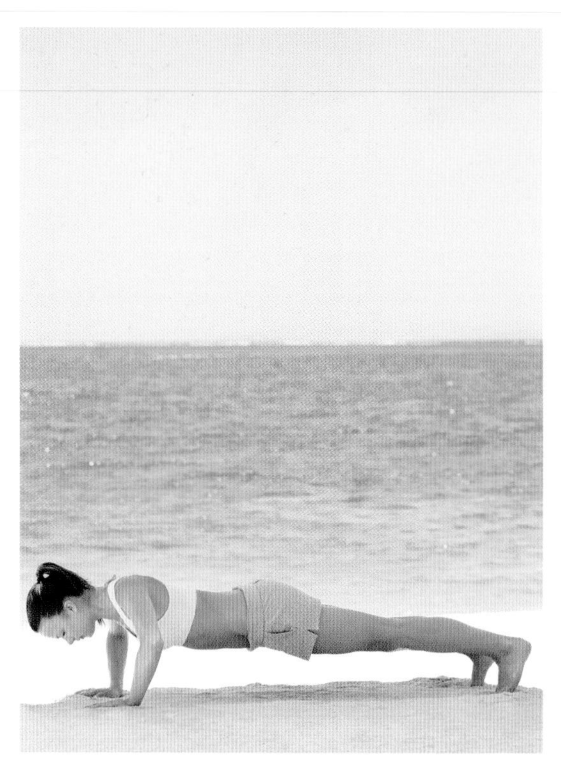

Push Up from Feet

How to do it

1 Set hands one and a half shoulder widths apart and in line with your nipples, NOT your shoulders, and legs straight with your weight distributed through the hands and toes.

2 Keep your ears, shoulders, and hips in alignment.

3 Contract your stomach muscles.

4 Lower yourself so your nose almost touches the ground, keeping your body straight, then lift back up to the start position.

5 Remember to keep your head up and belly button drawn in.

6 Breathe out as you push up to the start position, and breathe in as you lower yourself down.

*top tip

This strengthens your upper body and works your abdominals, plus it's a great way to tone your arms and chest.

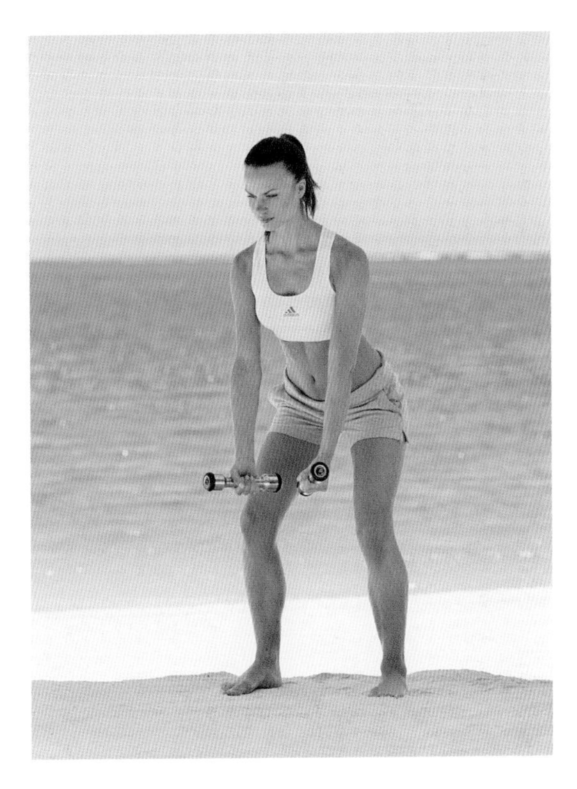

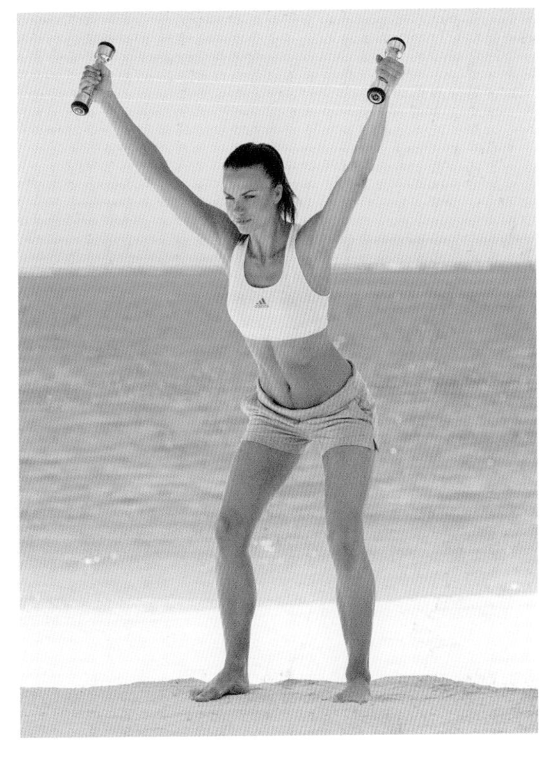

Weighted Y+T

How to do it

1 Standing up straight, bend your legs slightly and stick your bottom out.

2 Keep your back and head all in a straight line, with your shoulders down and back and keep the tummy tucked in.

3 Holding your weights in both hands, keeping your arms straight, bring both arms alongside your ears in a straight line making a "Y" shape.

4 Everything is the same with the "T," but bend down a little further and bring your arms to the side making a "T" shape.

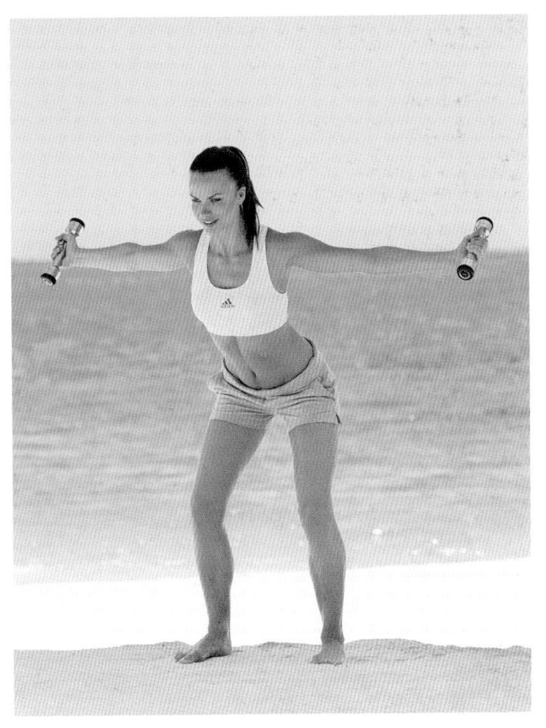

*top tip

Lack of grip strength can hinder your workout, so keep a squeeze ball in the car and work those hand muscles any chance you get.

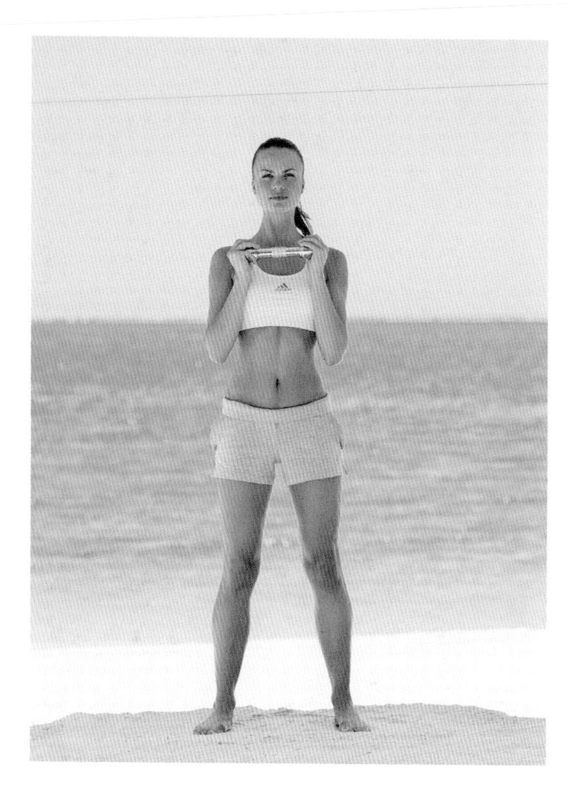

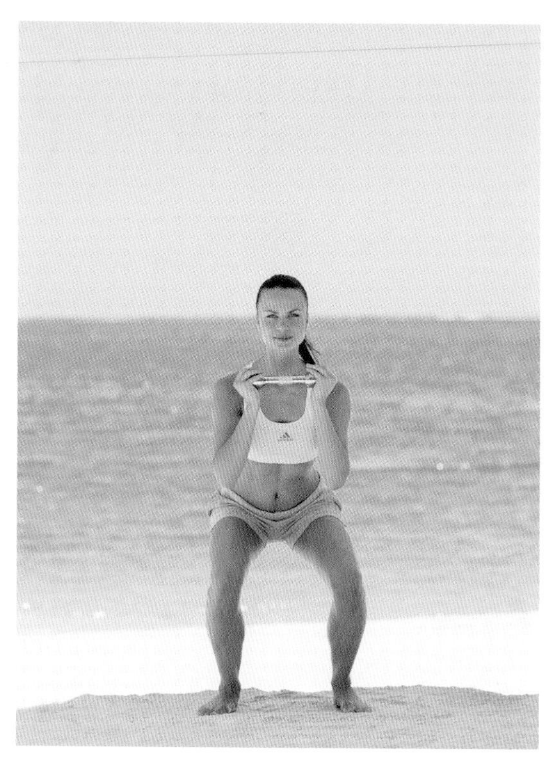

Push Press

How to do it

1 Stand while holding the weight at chest height.

2 Slowly squat down so your thighs are parallel to the floor.

3 As you come back to standing push your weights up over your head.

*top tip

This exercise works the legs, upper body and core.

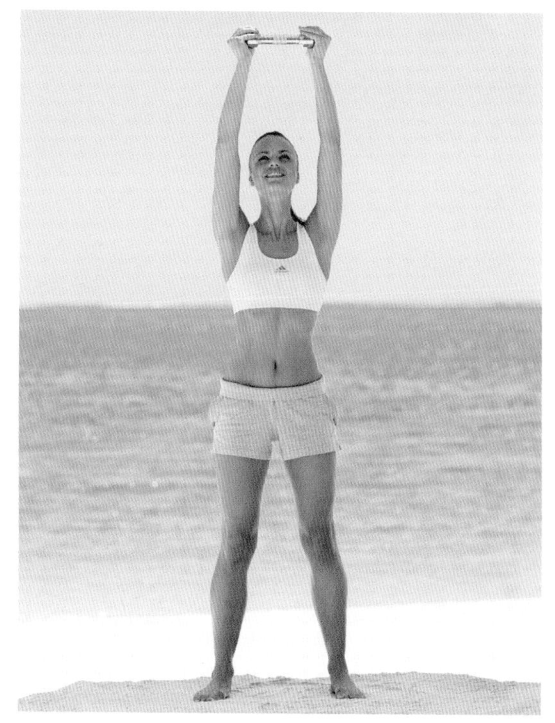

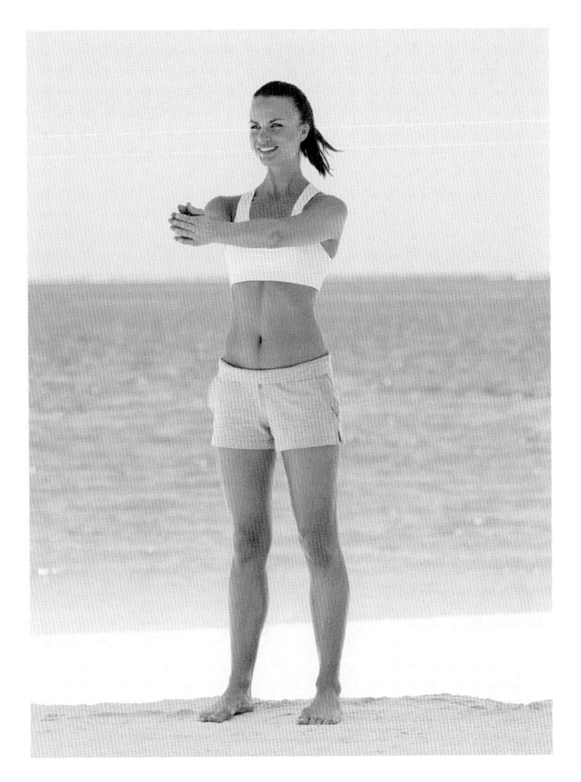

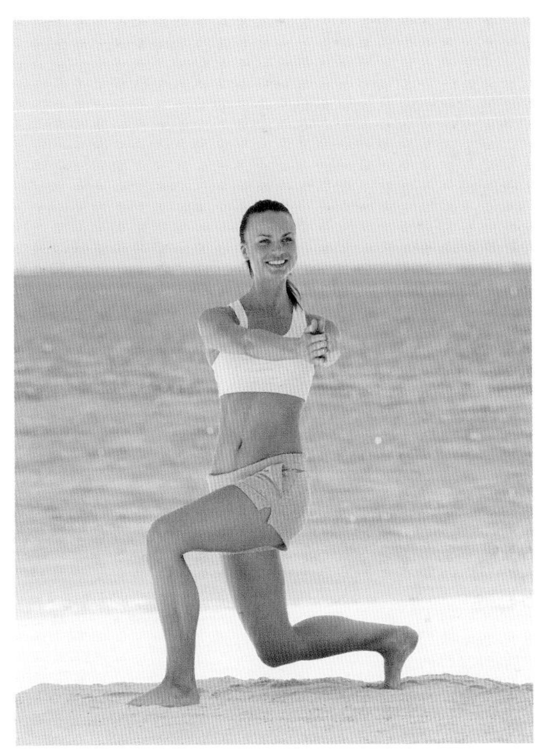

Dynamic Lunge with Rotation

How to do it

1 Stand up with perfect posture with palms facing outwards.
2 Both feet should face outwards.
3 Set the core.
4 Your feet should be hip-width apart.
5 Step forwards as shown. Your front shin should be straight and perpendicular to the floor.
6 Rotate your hips whilst maintaining core balance.
7 Push up with the front leg, returning to the standing position.

*top tip

This burns fat and helps improve balance.

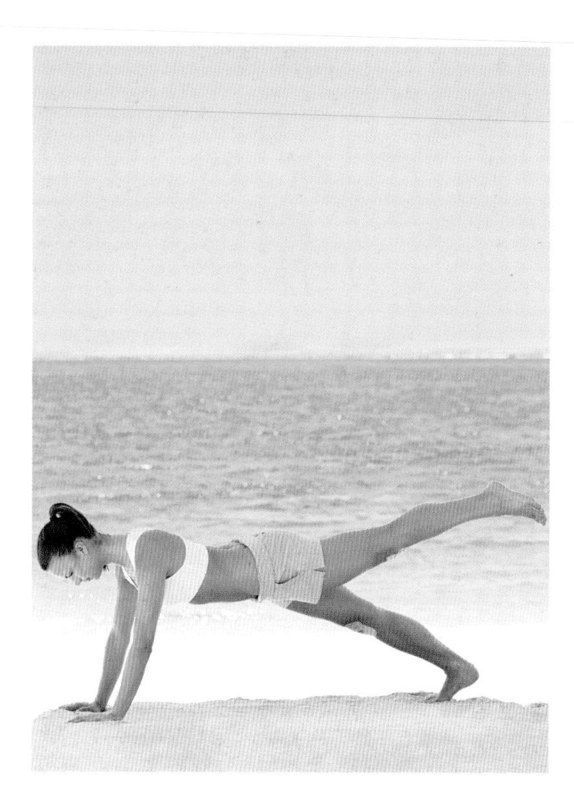

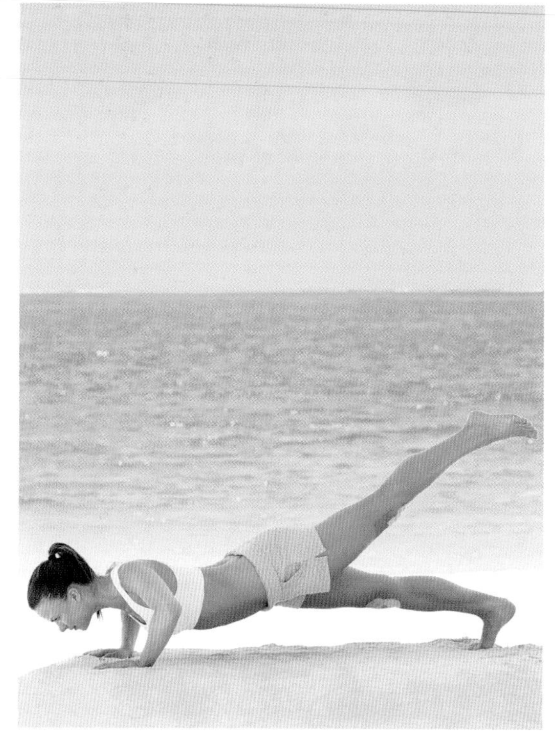

Single-legged Push Up

How to do it

1 Set your hands one and a half shoulder widths apart and in line with your nipples, NOT your shoulders.
2 Set perfect posture with your ears, shoulders, and hips in alignment.
3 Set the core.
4 Lower yourself for around 2 seconds keeping your body straight.
5 Remember to keep your head up and belly button drawn in.
6 Breath out as you push up to the start position.

*top tip

This strengthens your upper body and works your abdominals when done properly. It's also a great way to tone your arms and chest. By using only one leg the body is forced to use the stomach muscles more (to keep it steady).

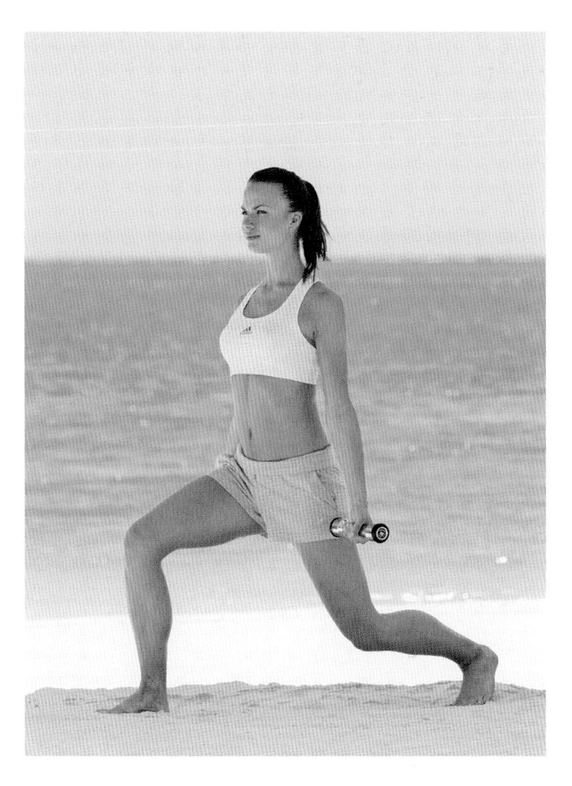

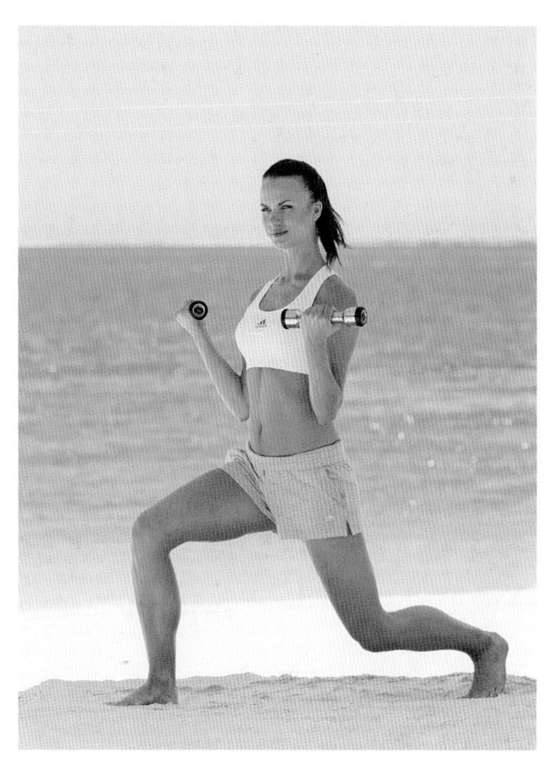

Split Squat with Bicep Curl

How to do it

1 Stand up with perfect posture with palms facing out. The feet should be hip-width apart and face forwards.
2 Set the core.
3 Position your feet as shown, with a straight front shin.
4 Hold the weights out as shown.
5 Lower your body by bending your back knee. The back knee should just touch the floor.
6 Push up, putting your weight through the heel of the front foot.
7 As you push up back to standing position complete a bicep curl as shown.

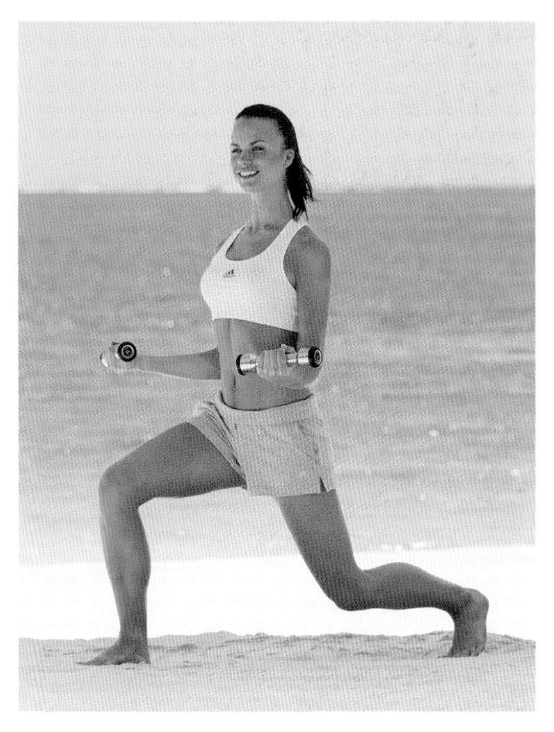

*top tip

This lunge is great for hitting your butt, hips and thighs. By adding the curl it works out your biceps too.

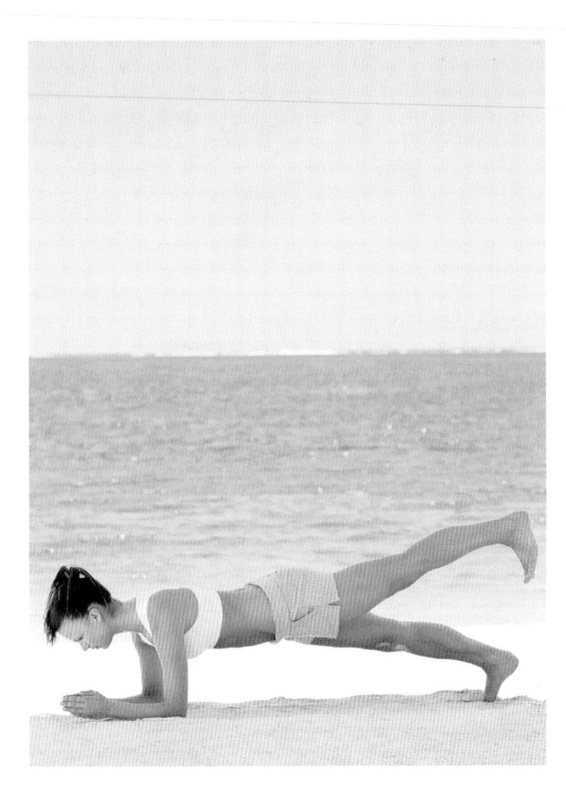

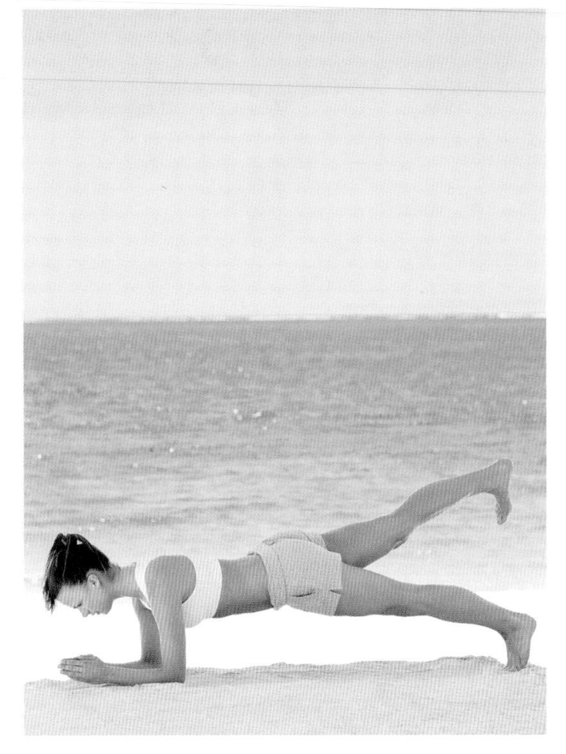

One-legged Plank

How to do it

1 Lie face down on the floor with forearms and elbows touching the floor, hips and legs on the ground.

2 Raise your hips and set the core, keeping your head aligned with your upper back and hips. Imagine a straight line from your head to your ankles.

3 Now lift one leg off the floor so the foot hovers about an inch off the floor and the hip stays level.

4 Hold your body off the floor.

*it's easy

For more programs, please go online to cleanandlean.com or bodyism.com.

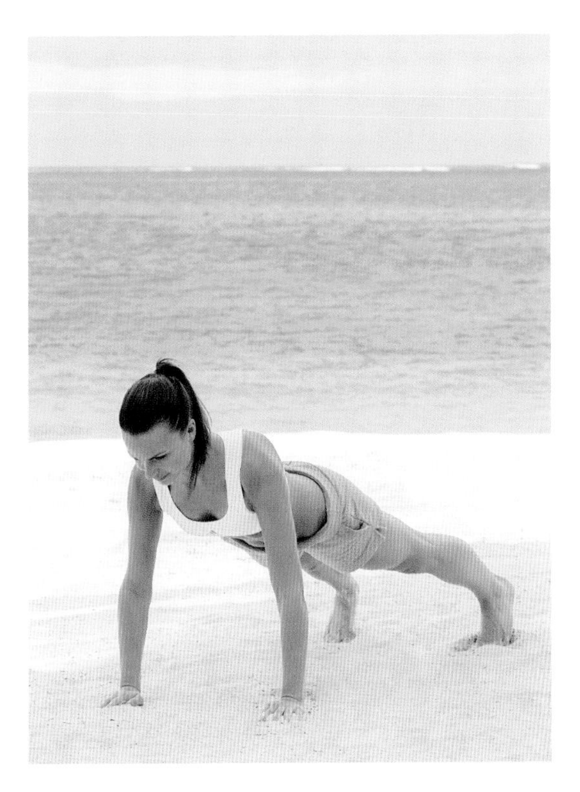

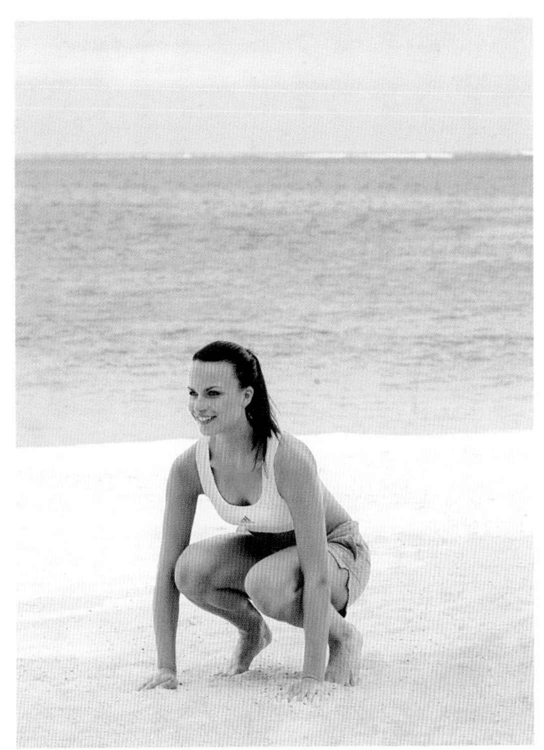

Burpie

How to do it

1 Start in a push up position with weight equally distributed between your hands and feet.

2 Jump your feet towards hands and then stand straight up with your hands in the air and then jump—as you land, ensure that the weight is equally distributed on each foot and that your landing is soft.

3 Once you have finished the jump then place your hands on the floor beside your feet and then jump your feet back into the original start position, keeping your back straight and abs tight.

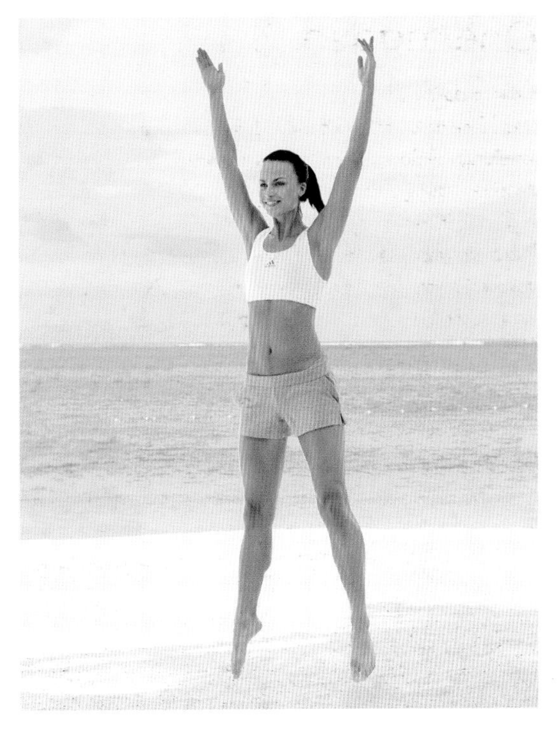

*top tip

This fantastic fat-burner is great for developing coordination with the upper and lower body and really working your legs and core.

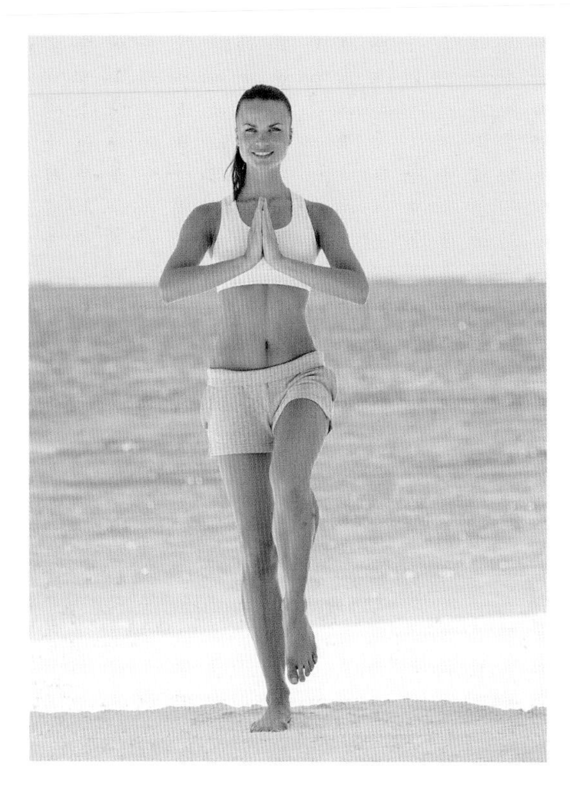
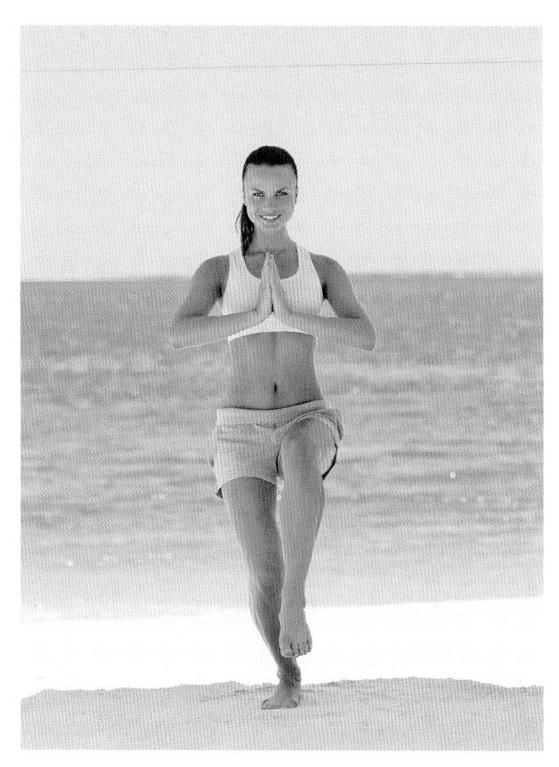

Single-legged Squat

How to do it

1 Set the core.
2 Take a comfortable stance, keeping your feet shoulder-width apart, or wider if necessary.
3 Join your hands and hold your arms parallel to the floor.
4 Point your toes out slightly and make sure your knees stay aligned with your second toe.
5 Lift one leg off the floor and squat down. DO NOT fall forwards when squatting.
6 Don't let the leg that is working buckle inwards.

*top tip

This is an excellent all-round exercise and is fantastic for your posture.

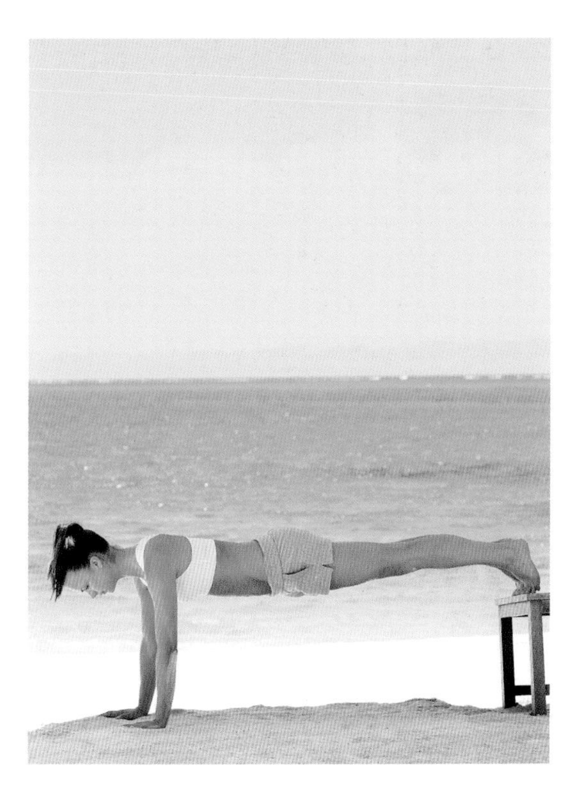

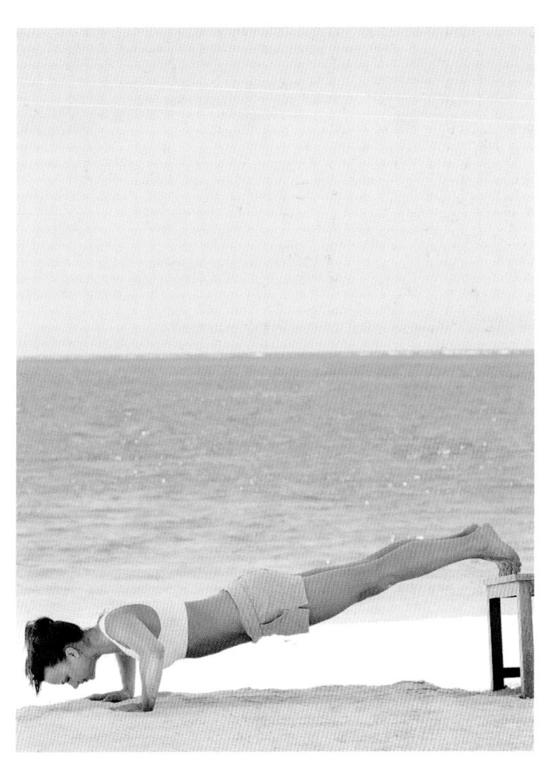

Push Ups with Elevated Feet

How to do it

1 Set hands one and a half shoulder widths apart and in line with your nipples, NOT your shoulders. Keep your legs straight with your weight distributed through your hands and toes.
2 Have your feet raised on either a step or sofa.
3 Keep your ears, shoulders, and hips in alignment.
4 Contract your stomach muscles.
5 Lower yourself so your nose almost touches the ground, keeping your body straight, then lift back up to the start position.
6 Remember to keep your head up and belly button drawn in.
7 Breathe out as you push up to start position, and breathe in as you lower yourself down.

*top tip

This strengthens your upper body and abdominals, and really works your arms and chest too. And with your feet raised it will work your abs even more!

Dynamic Lunge with Shoulder Press

How to do it

1 Stand up with perfect posture with palms facing outwards.
2 Both feet should face outwards.
3 Set the core.
4 Your feet should be hip-width apart.
5 Step forward as shown, bending your arms at the elbows. Your front shin should be straight and perpendicular to the floor.
6 Push up with the front leg, returning to the standing position.
7 As you come up, straighten your arms to lift the weights back up again.

*top tip

Adding a few extra movements burns even more fat as well as improving core balance.

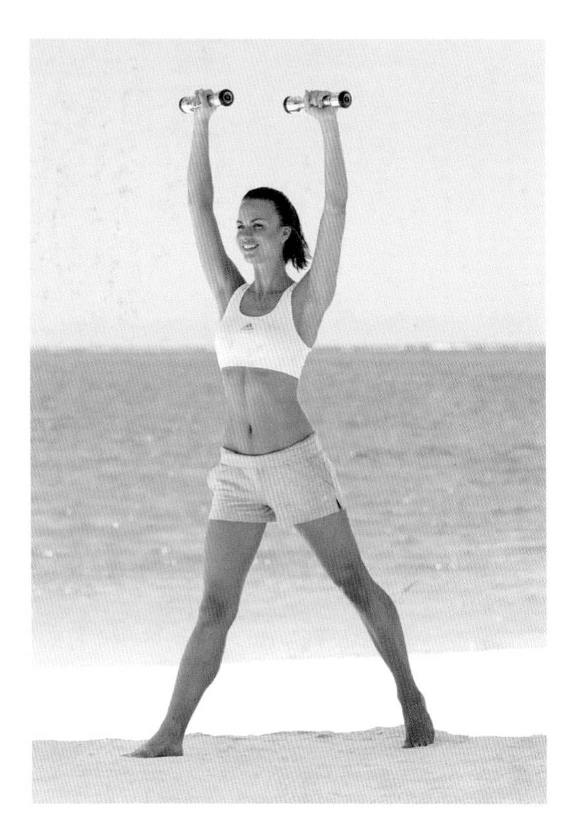

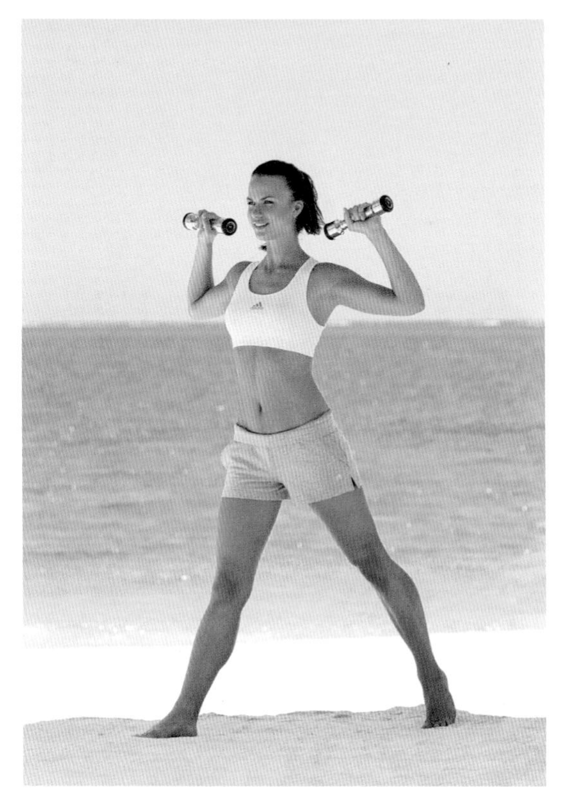

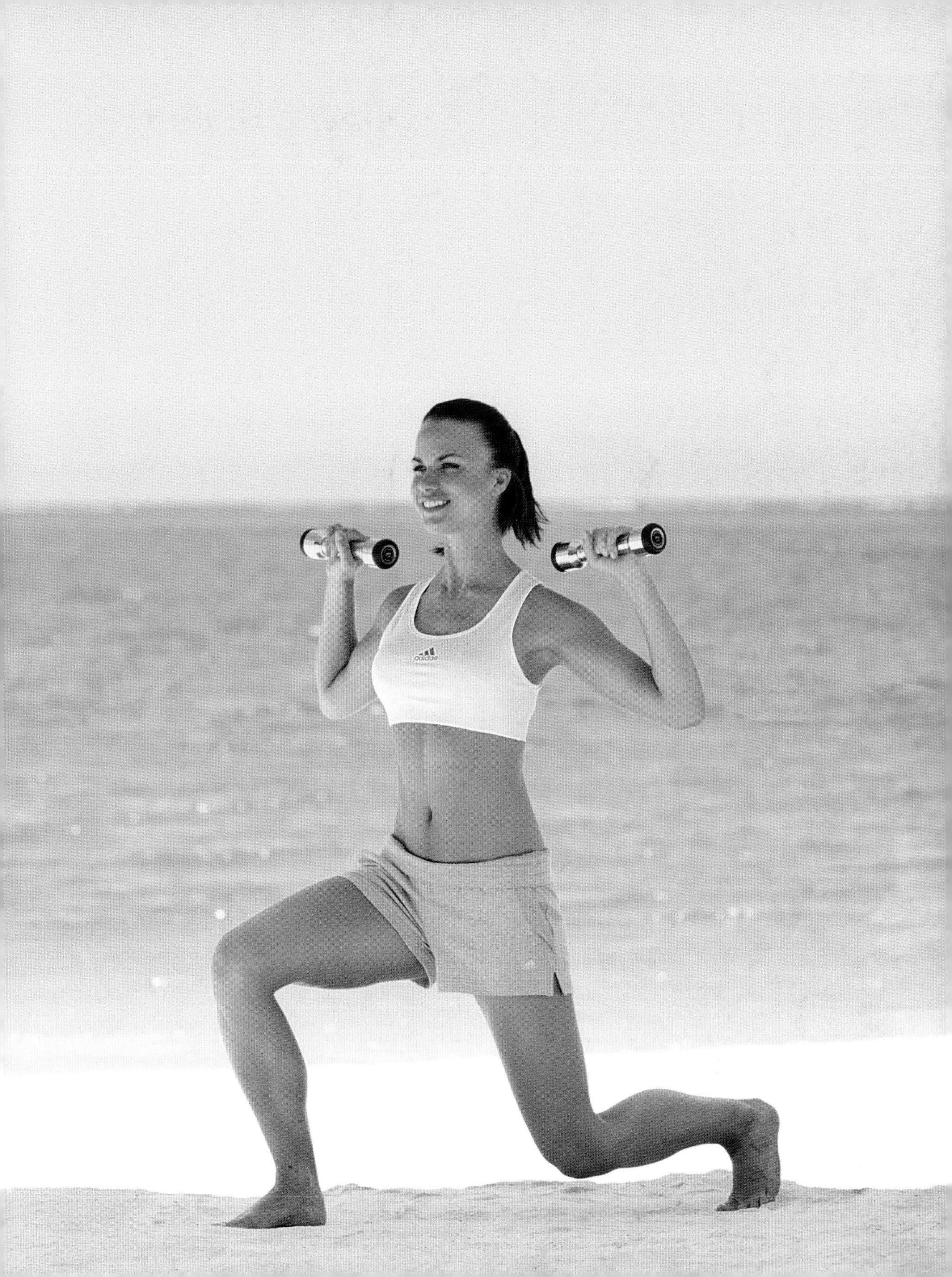
adidas

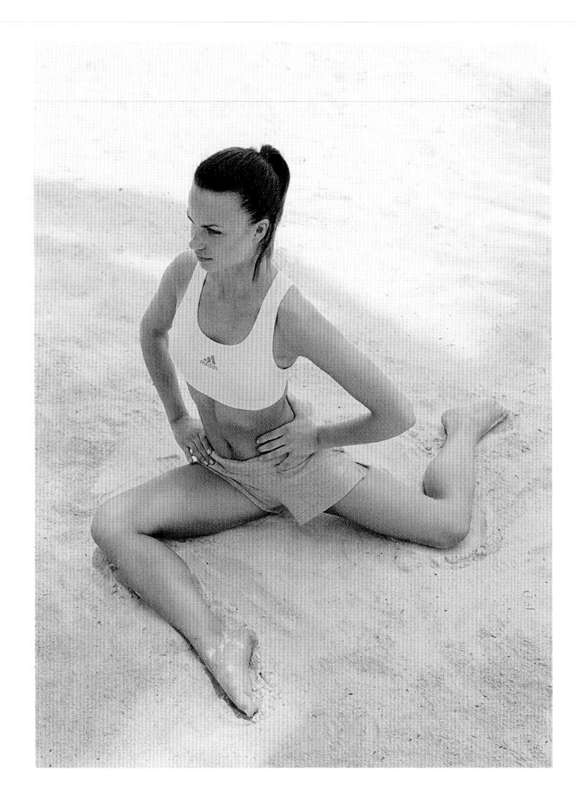

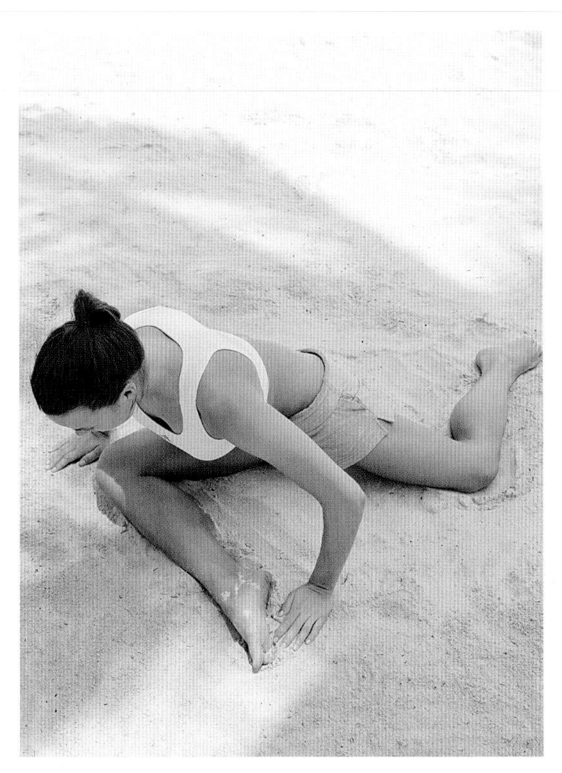

The Skinny Stretch

How to do it

1 Start off seated with the front leg bent at 90 degrees and back leg at 90 degrees.
2 Keeping your chest up, gently lean forwards, keeping a curve in your lower back.
3 You should feel a stretch in your hips and bottom.
4 Lean back and feel a stretch through the front of your thigh.
5 Raising your arm will increase the stretch and lengthen the muscle.
6 Hold the stretch for 10–15 seconds, then move out of the stretch, and repeat for the required number of repetitions.

*top tip

Remember to breath—your body will relax and you will be able to get a better stretch.

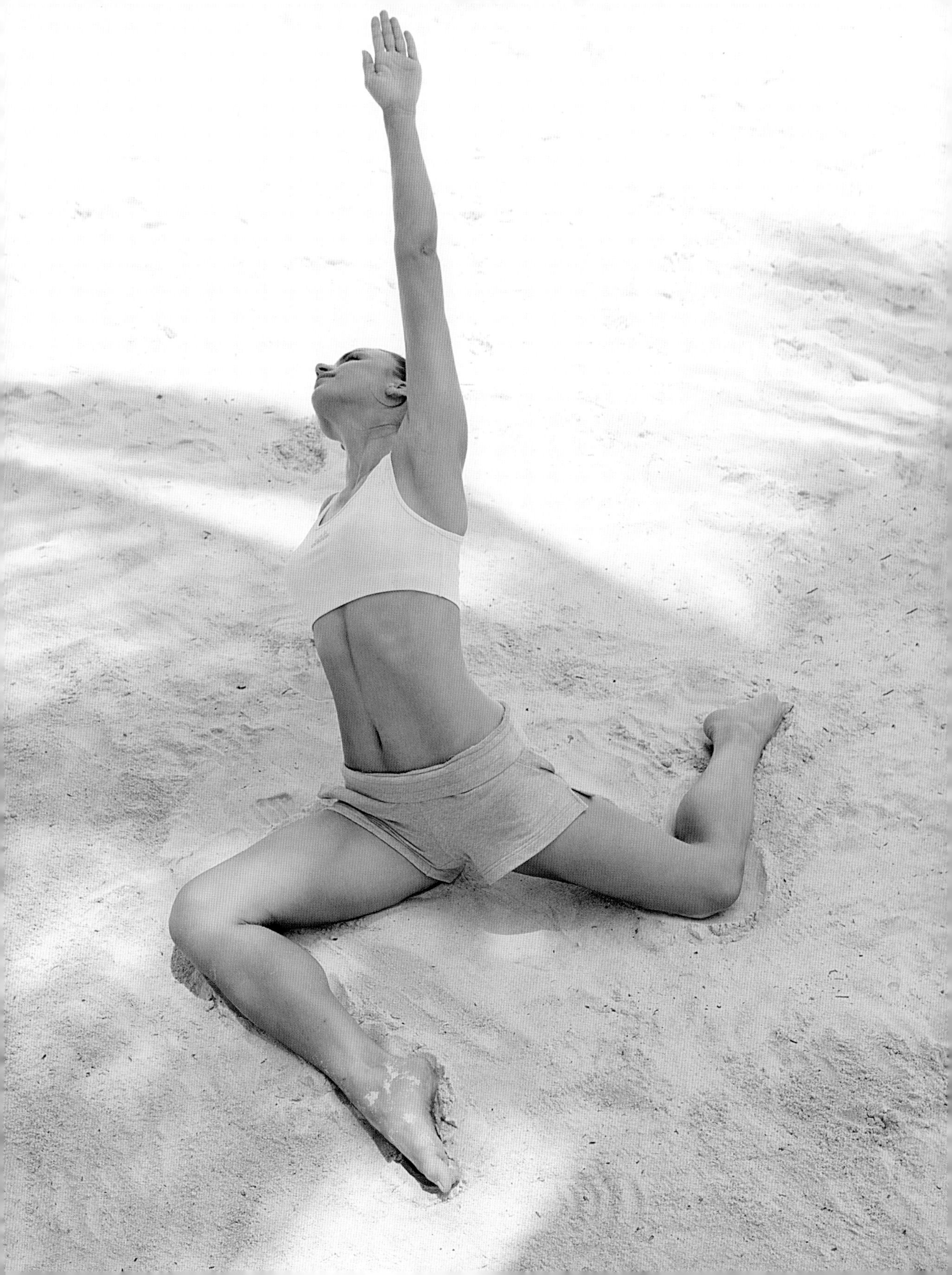

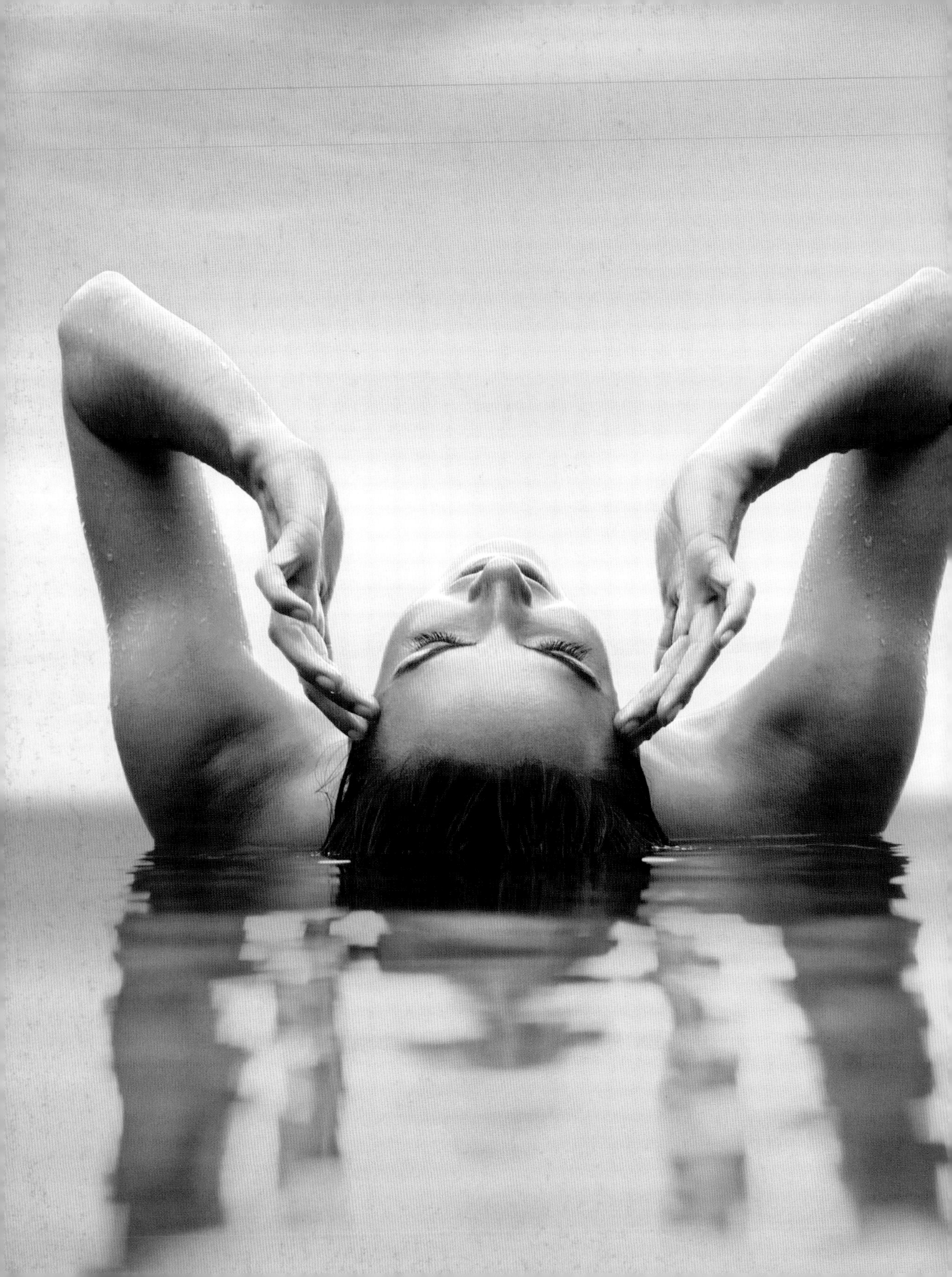

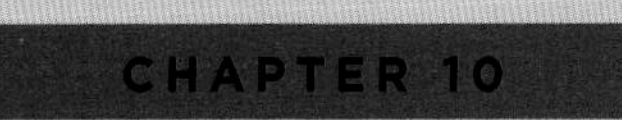

STAYING CLEAN & LEAN FOR LIFE

THIS CHAPTER WILL REVEAL...

A REMINDER OF THE CLEAN & LEAN BASICS

THE "CHEAT MEAL"

HOW NOT TO TALK YOURSELF TIRED

So you've got this far—well done! If you've followed my 14-day Clean & Lean Kickstart while reading the last nine chapters, you should be looking and feeling pretty amazing right now. But don't give it all up at this stage—because after the 14-day Kickstart I want you to stay Clean & Lean for life. This means making the recipes from my books and using what you've learned to select what works for you. It's easier than you'd imagine.

A REMINDER OF THE CLEAN & LEAN BASICS

I don't expect you to remember—or follow—every single thing I've recommended throughout this book. And I don't expect you to never have a glass of wine or a bar of chocolate ever again. In fact, I want you to have a blowout meal once a week (this is called a "cheat meal," and I'll explain more about that below). What I do want you to do more than anything is to follow the Clean & Lean basics. Here's a brief reminder:

✳ Choose clean, lean foods and drinks as much as possible. Whether you're shopping for food, or selecting from a menu, always go for the cleanest, most natural-looking food or meal you see. If you can't recognize a food or its contents, give it a miss.
✳ Avoid sugar at all costs—there really are no benefits. So next time you're tempted by a pretty pink cupcake, think again.
✳ Eat plenty of good fats—they will take years off your face, banish cravings and help to slim down your waist.
✳ Exercise at least three times a week—even if you just do my 8-minute plan.
✳ Cut back on alcohol.
✳ Don't stress-eat.
✳ When in doubt, eat fish and greens! Think, Lean and Green!
✳ Stress makes you fat—chill out and you'll lose weight.
✳ Stick to two coffees a day—maximum!

DON'T TALK YOURSELF TIRED/ FAT/TOXIC

Half the battle when it comes to keeping your body in shape is keeping your mind in shape too. I once spent an entire year being tired without even realizing that I was causing the whole problem myself. I was working hard and training harder, and whenever anybody asked me how I was, my automatic response would be: "I'm exhausted." Pretty soon my body started believing what I was constantly telling it.

Then, one day, my best friend and I were having lunch and he asked how I was. As usual I replied, "I'm completely shattered." He just shook his head and told me I'd been giving him the same answer for a year and that it was becoming boring. This hit me like a slap in the face. I'd been talking myself into feeling tired for a whole year! From that second on, I promised myself that I wouldn't tell anyone—including myself—that I was tired or exhausted. When somebody asked me how I felt I'd say, "Amazing, thanks!" That message started filtering into my body and I really did start to feel amazing.

So don't describe yourself as tired, or fat or unfit. You can feel amazing, you can feel energized and you can feel slim and fit. You just have to change your attitude.

*top tip

Be kind to yourself. Remember that a transformation in your body, happens in your mind first. You DO deserve a healthy, happy life. Understand the power of your thoughts and words and no more negative talking or thinking.

The "Cheat Meal"

I tell all my clients to have a "cheat meal" once a week, at which they can eat anything they like. (At my own weekly cheat meal I tuck into hot chocolate pudding with ice cream!) This helps to keep you on track, and it also helps you lose weight (believe it or not). This is because when you're following a good, healthy diet all the time, your metabolism stays steady. However, when you eat more than usual, your metabolism goes into shock and starts working overtime to burn off the extra food. Of course, if you eat this way all the time, your metabolism will get used to it and your body will just store—and get—fat. But if you do it just once a week your metabolism stays sky high. Plus it keeps you on the diet bandwagon because you know where your next treat is coming from and don't feel deprived. So make sure you enjoy the hell out of your cheat meal and choose the tastiest thing you can find. As I always say: "If you're going to be bad, make it damned good!"

LAUREN'S STORY

"I found James and the Clean & Lean diet in a vain attempt to look like Rosie Huntington-Whiteley (can you blame me?!), but what I found was far more powerful than I could have ever imagined. James taught me about the effect of food on your general wellbeing but the most life changing part of the Clean & Lean philosophy for me is the importance of self-love, reducing stress and banning negative self-talk. For the first time in my life I am building a strong body as well as a strong mind. Clean & Lean has truly given me a new lease on life."

And Finally

Here's your final Bad, Better and Best table. Use it as a general guide in everyday life to help you make the cleanest, leanest choices possible (or refer back to my previous ones, for more specific issues).

BAD	BETTER	BEST
Peanut butter—contains hydrogenated fats and sugar	**Organic peanut butter**—a good source of vitamin E, without the bad trans fats	**Organic nut butter** (e.g. almond, cashew or macadamia)—full of healthy fats and antioxidants
Muffin—full of sugar and bad fats	**Fruit and nuts**—natural sugars and protein will leave you far more satisfied	**Super Skinny Smoothie** (see p. 121)
Skim milk—with no fat, the body cannot absorb calcium in milk	**Organic full-fat milk**—contains fewer harmful fats than the non-organic type	**Organic goat milk**—easier to digest and naturally higher in Vitamin A and B
Flavored yogurt—full of sugar and heavily processed	**Organic flavored yogurt**—natural ingredients, but still high in sugar	**Organic full-fat natural yogurt with nuts**—no artificial flavoring, and the protein in the nuts makes it a complete and satisfying snack
White bread—heavily processed, with little nutritional value	**Rye bread**—higher in fiber and much tastier	**Rice bread**—gluten-free, this won't leave you feeling bloated
Chips or fries—cooked in fat and low in nutritional value	**Wedges with guacamole**—baking or roasting wedges is healthier, and the guacamole contains good fats	**Baked sweet potato with meat/ tuna**—the healthiest option, with a good serving of protein
Tinned fish—nutrients are lost during the canning process	**Fresh fish**—fresh is always better, but farmed fish may contain chemicals picked up from their diet	**Wild organic fish**—natural, unprocessed, and full of essential proteins and fatty acids
Sandwich—might fill you up, but the wheat in the bread may leave you bloated and sluggish	**Spelt sandwich with chicken and tomato salsa**—higher in fiber nutrients than a regular sandwich	**Clean & Lean chicken lettuce wraps**—gluten-free and full of nutrients
Deep-fried food	**Pan-fried food**—uses less fat	**Grilled, steamed or boiled food**—the best option, completely avoiding cooking fat
Microwave meal—pre-packed meals are often highly processed and microwaving can kill nutrients	**Pre-packaged meal heated in oven**—still not as good as freshly prepared food but the oven is a better cooking method	**Chicken stir-fry with five types of vegetables**—the perfect high-nutrient, low-calorie meal

BAD	BETTER	BEST
Hamburger and fries—processed meat, fatty fries, and the wheat in the bun may leave you feeling bloated	**Hamburger and sweet potato fries**—these fries are richer in nutrients than a bun	**Grass-fed beef patty and salad**—grass-fed offers protein and higher omega-3's and isn't heavily processed
Battered fish—coating is fatty, and often deep-fried	**Pan-fried fish with salad**—better than deep fried, battered fish, and the salad makes a healthier meal	**Steamed wild fish and salad**—the healthiest option, you should eat this regularly
Chicken nuggets—heavily processed, high in salt and bad fats	**BBQ chicken and salad**—better than nuggets, but BBQ sauces are often full of sugar	**Grilled free-range chicken with salsa, spinach, and avocado** (see p. 94)
Pre-packaged garlic bread—often poor-quality bread, and will contain artificial flavorings	**Homemade garlic bread** (crush some garlic on to bread and grill with olive oil)—natural and delicious	**Garlic mashed with olive oil and peppers**—lose the bread completely
Packaged tortellini—processed and often contains artificial flavorings	**Pasta with meat sauce**—homemade and a good source of protein	**Wheat-free pasta with Clean & Lean Super Ground Beef Sauce** (see p. 111)
Jello—full of sugar and artificial flavoring	**Jello with fruit**—still too much sugar but at least the fruit offers some nutrients	**Fruit with nuts**—ideally berries—a natural source of sugar, with protein to fill you up
Ice cream—full of sugar and the milk is hard to digest	**Organic ice cream**—free of pesticides, synthetic hormones, and antibiotics. Much less toxic	**Organic cashew nut ice cream**—a dairy-free alternative that contains healthy fats, protein, and carbohdrates
Strawberry jam—full of high-GI sugar with little fiber content	**Peanut butter**—a good source of healthy fats, fiber, and protein	**Organic nut butter**—pesticide-free and a source of healthy fats and fiber
Runny honey—no fiber, very little nutrient content and causes a big rise in blood sugar levels	**Manuka honey**—natural antibacterial, antimicrobial, antiseptic, antiviral, antioxidant, anti-inflammatory, and antifungal properties	**Organic raw honey**—a natural sweetener that has antibiotic properties
Crackers with packaged pâté—just baked flour with no nutritional value, and packaged pâté may be full of preservatives and artificial flavorings	**Crackers with freshly made deli pâté**—freshly made doesn't contain as much salt or preservatives	**Sweet potato crackers with homemade hummus**—hummus is high in protein and sweet potato is low-GI and nutrient-rich
Artificial sweetener	**Brown sugar**—marginally higher nutritional value than white sugar	**Manuka honey and a squeeze of lemon**—contains some nutrients

{INDEX}

{INDEX}

{ACKNOWLEDGMENTS}

I am so grateful to so many people, I can't fit them all on one page but here goes. To my wife and best friend, Chrissy. I love you so much, you're everything that's good in our world. To our little girl Charlotte, we love everything about you, every second of every day. You saved your grandpa's life by giving him the best reason in the world to live. To Tom Konig for being the best man in the world and for being so unbelievably kind to us. To Rosie H-W for being so wonderful to me, you're truly amazing and have always been there for us no matter what. To David de Rothschild for being a constant source of inspiration and strength, and for being Charlotte's godfather and teaching her to be kind and curious and anything but normal. Knowing people like you are in the world makes me smile. To Theresa Palmer, a friend straight from heaven to bring magic and babies into our lives. You met Charlotte even before we did, she couldn't ask for a better god-mummy. To Lee and Nat, you stood by us through everything and now we're really having fun! We love you guys so much. Lee Mullins—male model/DJ/Eastenders actor and semi-pro footballer, you have been a better friend than I could ever have hoped for. I've watched you grow into one of the finest and most brilliant men I've ever had the privileged to know. Nat, you are amazing, brilliant, loyal, and most of all a wonderful friend to us—it was you who helped us rebuild Bodyism better than ever. To my friends for being my strength and loving me, especially Mike, Justin, Lee, and Ben. To the incomparable Stephanie Haynes, you continue to bless us with kindness and love and Tom is just too stylish. Hani, we will always remember that you saved us. Vincent, I'm just glad you're on our side! Ivan and Marina for giving me a place to write these books and make beautiful babies. Luke, Chantal, Sienna, and Jake, all world champions. Tatiana, for being a truer friend than we could have ever hoped for. Mandy Ferry, you are an angel to us. Elle, thanks for teaching me that a true friend will stick with you through thick and thin. To Joe Dowdell for standing with us and being such an amazing support. To Jamie Wendt, for driving this thing and parking? To Ruby, Auntie do-lots. To our wonderful, amazing parents, Stella, Helo, Peter, and Kevin—thank you for loving us and supporting us; we are blessed to have the most wonderful family in the world and we owe you everything. To Josh Stolz for your giant brain and your giant heart. Edwina, Jess, and Loz, not for one moment did you leave us and we'll always remember and always love you. Deborah Arthurs, you are the best. To Maria, I can't believe you did it again! To my long-suffering publishers, thank you for your patience and flexible deadlines. To the Clean & Lean community, you are an amazing group of people and you are the reason I am able to write these books. The Bodyism team, for now, truly being the best in the world and making everything so wonderful. To Hugh Grant for being my friend and for having integrity and being kind and fabulous in your panties. And thank you God, I prayed to you when I had no hope and I promised I wouldn't ignore you anymore, thanks for being there for me always.

It will all be OK in the end, and if it's not OK, it's not the end.

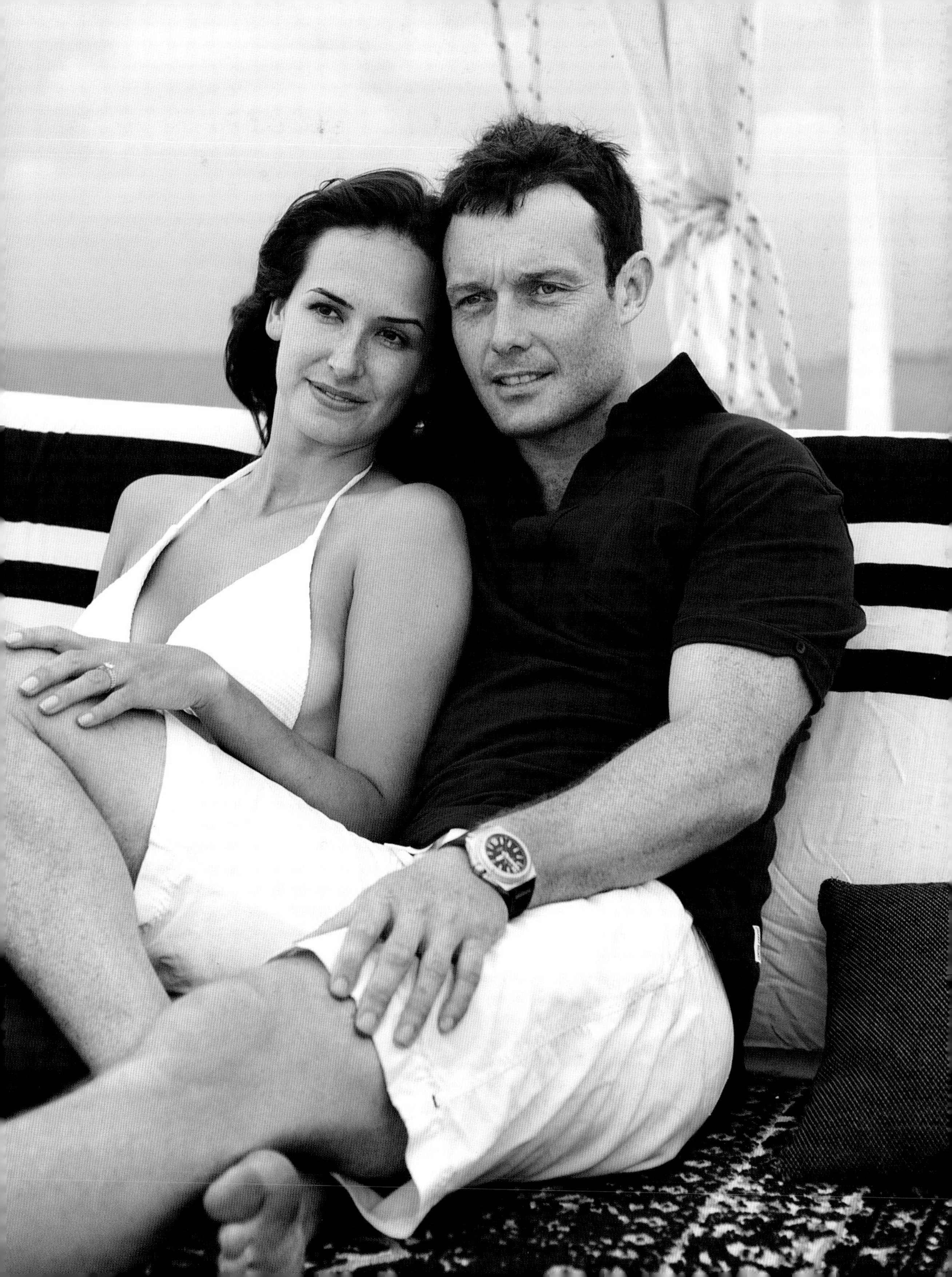

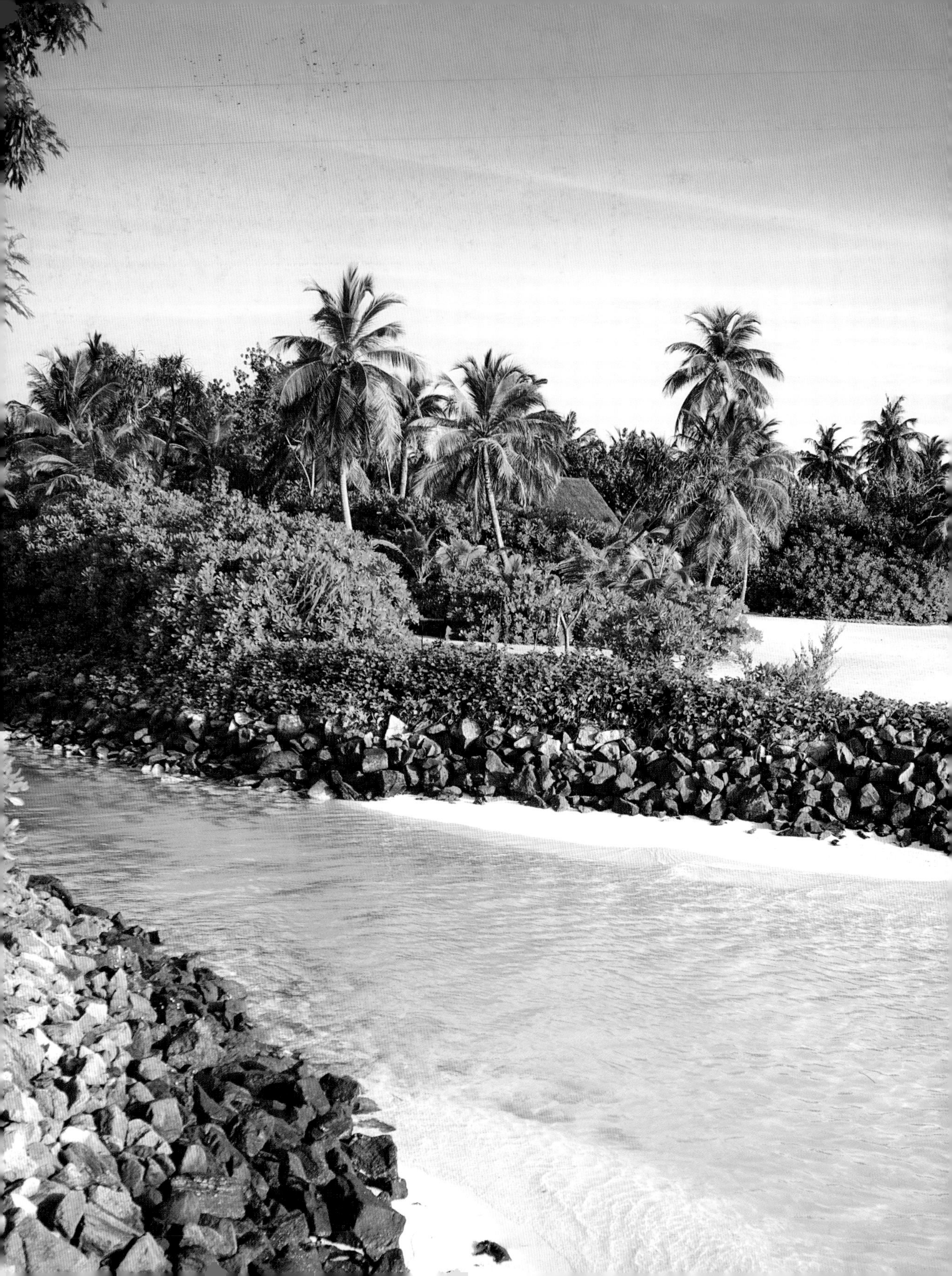